ANATOMY FOR

ARM BALANCES

AND

INVERSIONS

RAY LONG, MD, FRCSC

bandha yoga publications

This book is intended as a reference volume only, not as a medical manual. It is not to be used in any manner for diagnosis or treatment of medical or surgical conditions. This book is also not intended to be a substitute for any treatment that may be or has been prescribed by your health care provider. If you suspect that you have a medical problem, consult your physician. Always, in your particular case, obtain medical clearance from your physician before beginning the practice of yoga or any other exercise program. Always practice yoga under the direct guidance and supervision of a qualified and experienced instructor. Working directly with a qualified yoga instructor can help to prevent injuries. The author, illustrators, editor, publisher and distributor specifically disclaim any responsibility or liability for injuries that may occur during the practice of yoga or any other exercise program.

Published by Bandha Yoga Publications
Plattsburgh, NY
www.bandhayoga.com

Distributed by Greenleaf Book Group LLC

For ordering information and bulk purchases, contact Bandha Yoga Publications.
info@bandhayoga.com
Phone: 518.578.3720

Design and composition by Greenleaf Book Group LLC
Cover design by Greenleaf Book Group LLC
Front and back cover illustrations by Kurt Long, BFA www.kurtlong.net
Computer Graphics Technical Director: Chris Macivor
Sanskrit calligraphy and border painting: Stewart Thomas www.palmstone.com
Editor: Eryn Kirkwood, MA, RYT www.barrhavenyoga.com

ISBN 13: 978-1-60743-945-5

Part of the Tree Neutral™ program, which offsets the number of trees consumed in the production and printing of this book by taking proactive steps, such as planting trees in direct proportion to the number of trees used: www.treeneutral.com

Printed in China on acid-free paper

10 11 12 13 14 15 10 9 8 7 6 5 4 3 2 1

First Edition

CONTENTS

INTRODUCTION

THE MAT COMPANION SERIES PROVIDES A METHODICAL APPROACH FOR USING science to balance and connect the body and mind in yoga. The fourth book concludes the series with arm balances and inversions—two pose categories that clearly integrate opposites within the body.

In our bipedal form, the hips and lower extremities are the weight-bearing construct. The more mobile shoulders and upper extremities allow us to interact with the world. In arm balances, we invert this construct, thereby strengthening the muscles, bones, and ligaments of the upper extremities. From an energetic perspective, arm balances stimulate the nerve plexuses associated with the fourth and fifth chakras. Practicing these poses with precision moves nerve impulses upwards through the subtle body. This opens the way for the unimpeded flow of energy from the lower and more primordial regions of the sacral plexus to the higher-functioning levels of the brain.

A similar balancing of opposites takes place with inverted poses. Consider that most of our time is spent with the head above the heart and the lower extremities below it. Inversions reverse this, bringing the head below the heart and the lower extremities above it. Potential benefits of this body position include lowered blood pressure and heart rate and improved circulation of endorphins in the brain. All of this prepares the body for deep relaxation.

Arm balances invigorate and stimulate the mind. Inversions bring it to rest.

HOW TO USE THIS BOOK

Practicing yoga is like passing through a series of doors, with each door revealing new possibilities in the poses. The key to unlocking the first door is understanding the joint positions. This understanding can be used to identify the muscles that create the form of the pose and those that stretch. The key to positioning the joints is engaging the correct muscles. This begins with the prime movers. Engage the prime movers and the bones will align. The key to deepening the asanas is using your understanding of physiology to lengthen the muscles that stretch in the pose. Focus on these keys and the postures will automatically fall into place and manifest the beneficial effects of yoga. These include improved flexibility, heightened awareness, a sense of well-being, and deep relaxation.

The Mat Companion series is a set of modular books. Each book focuses on a specific pose category and contains the following:

- **The Key Concepts:** a description of biomechanical and physiological principles with applications for specific poses.
- **The Bandha Yoga Codex:** a simple five-step process that can be used to improve your flexibility, strength, and precision in the asanas.
- **The Pose Section:** a detailed description of the individual postures.
- **Movement Index:** explanations of body movement and tables listing the muscles associated with each movement.
- **Anatomy Index:** a visual listing of bones, ligaments, and muscles (showing the origins, insertions, and actions of each).
- **Glossary of Terms**
- **Sanskrit Pronunciation and Pose Index**
- **English Pose Index**

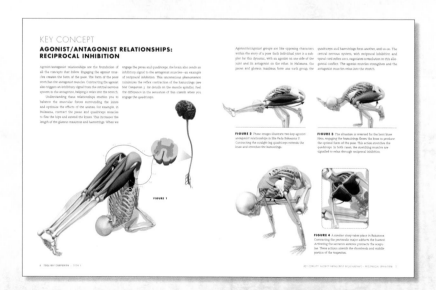

FIGURE 1 The Key Concepts show you how to apply biomechanics and physiology to your poses. Read this section first and return here often to refresh your knowledge.

FIGURE 2 The opening page for each pose illustrates the basic joint actions and positions of the body for that particular asana. Sanskrit and English names are provided for each posture. Use this page to assist you in learning the basic form of the pose and other concise details.

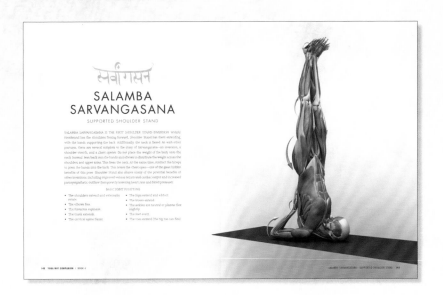

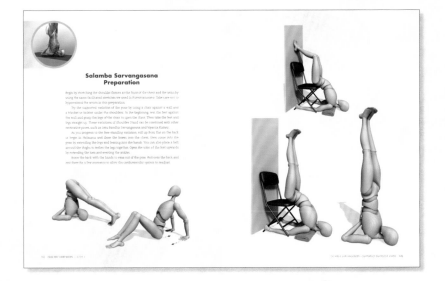

FIGURE 3 Use the preparatory section as a guide for how to enter the pose. If you are new to yoga or feel a bit stiff, use one of these modifications for your practice. In general, the preparatory poses affect the same muscle groups as the final asana. You will benefit from the pose no matter which variation you practice.

FIGURE 4 Each pose comes with a series of steps for engaging the muscles that position the joints, concluding with a summary of the muscles that stretch. Muscles that contract are colored different shades of blue (with the prime movers deep blue), and those that stretch are red. Use the pose section to master the anatomy of any given asana.

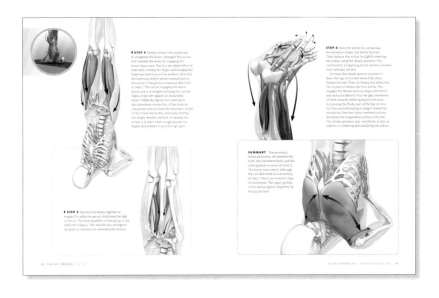

EVERY POSE TELLS A STORY

Paintings, sculptures, and yoga poses—like written works or cinema—all tell a story. With this in mind, it is helpful to look at the elements that create a narrative and see how they can be used to benefit your practice. Central to any story is a conflict that must be reconciled or an obstacle that must be overcome. Tension builds, and a crescendo is reached, followed by denouement. A solution must be negotiated. In the best stories, this dynamic evokes a cognitive shift in the audience, a new perspective. Consider this in the context of a pose or practice session. Use the metaphor of narrative structure to deepen the transformative power of yoga.

Let's deconstruct the story of Downward Facing Dog: contracting the psoas and its synergists flexes the hips and trunk. The hip extensors oppose this action, creating a conflict or obstacle. Increasing the contractile force of the psoas builds tension, which the gluteus maximus, its antagonist, resists. Sensory receptors relay information to the spinal cord about the muscle's length and tension. The central nervous system then negotiates a solution to the conflict through reciprocal inhibition and other physiological processes. The stretching muscle relaxes, the metaphorical obstacle is overcome, and the body moves deeper into the pose. Endorphins are released, producing a general sense of well-being and emotional balance. The lower chakras associated with the sacral plexus are stimulated, and energetic openings occur within the subtle body. A multilayered cognitive shift takes place.

We then move our attention to another subplot of the main story. Understanding that the main story of Dog Pose is a focused stretch of the hamstrings and gluteals, we can call on supporting cast to amplify this. In Downward Facing Dog, this means contracting the triceps. This force is transmitted to the lower extremities, as the torso is pressed back toward the thighs. We can also shift the focus to an agonist/antagonist group such as the quadriceps and hamstrings, repeating the process described above for the hip flexors. As the intensity of the stretch increases, the conflict escalates, until finally a crescendo is reached when the posture is complete. We move to the next posture, using the breath to weave the practice together.

It is said that the conscious mind cannot focus on more than two objects at one time. When we synchronize our attention on the breath and individual muscle groups, we eliminate mental chatter and cultivate a state of meditative absorption, all the while sculpting the pose.

KEY
CONCEPTS

KEY CONCEPT
AGONIST/ANTAGONIST RELATIONSHIPS: RECIPROCAL INHIBITION

Agonist/antagonist relationships are the foundation of all the concepts that follow. Engaging the agonist muscles creates the form of the pose. The form of the pose stretches the antagonist muscles. Contracting the agonist also triggers an inhibitory signal from the central nervous system to the antagonist, helping it relax into the stretch.

Understanding these relationships enables you to balance the muscular forces surrounding the joints and optimize the effects of the asanas. For example, in Halasana, contract the psoas and quadriceps muscles to flex the hips and extend the knees. This increases the length of the gluteus maximus and hamstrings. When we engage the psoas and quadriceps, the brain also sends an inhibitory signal to the antagonist muscles—an example of reciprocal inhibition. This unconscious phenomenon minimizes the reflex contraction of the hamstrings (see *Mat Companion 3* for details on the muscle spindle). Feel the difference in the sensation of this stretch when you engage the quadriceps.

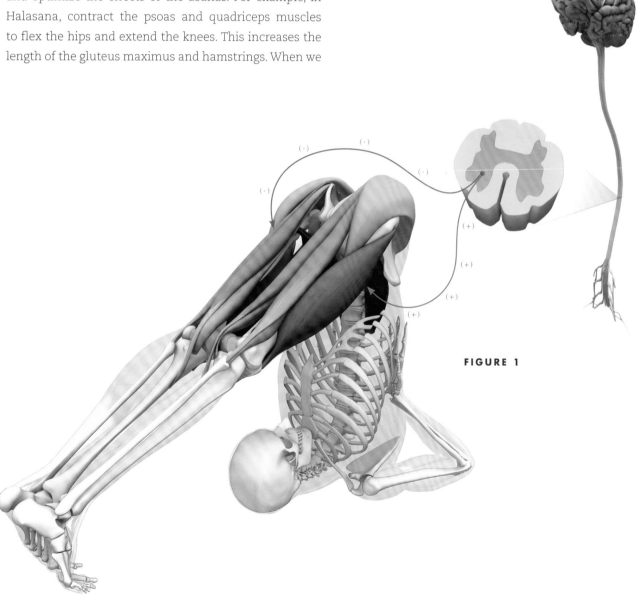

FIGURE 1

Agonist/antagonist groups are like opposing characters within the story of a pose. Each individual joint is a sub-plot for this dynamic, with an agonist on one side of the joint and its antagonist on the other. In Halasana, the psoas and gluteus maximus form one such group, the quadriceps and hamstrings form another, and so on. The central nervous system, with reciprocal inhibition and spinal cord reflex arcs, negotiates a resolution to this allegorical conflict. The agonist muscles strengthen and the antagonist muscles relax into the stretch.

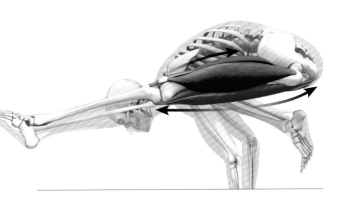

FIGURE 2 These images illustrate two key agonist/antagonist relationships in Eka Pada Bakasana II. Contracting the straight-leg quadriceps extends the knee and stretches the hamstrings.

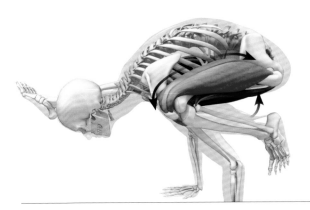

FIGURE 3 The situation is reversed for the bent knee. Here, engaging the hamstrings flexes the knee to produce the optimal form of the pose. This action stretches the quadriceps. In both cases, the stretching muscles are signalled to relax through reciprocal inhibition.

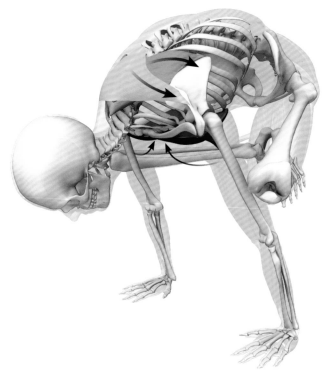

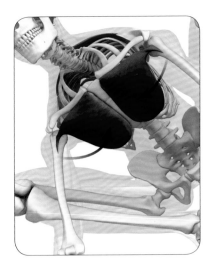

FIGURE 4 A similar story takes place in Bakasana. Contracting the pectoralis major adducts the humeri. Activating the serratus anterior protracts the scapulae. These actions stretch the rhomboids and middle portion of the trapezius.

KEY CONCEPT
KEY MUSCLE ISOLATIONS

Muscle isolation focuses your mental camera on one character and in the process sculpts one region of the asana. Isolating a muscle also stimulates both the sensory and motor neurons associated with that muscle and its antagonist group. "Walking" around the body by progressively isolating different muscle groups (as laid out in the steps for each pose) produces an imprint of the asana on the brain. Precisely positioning the joints brings this mental image into focus.

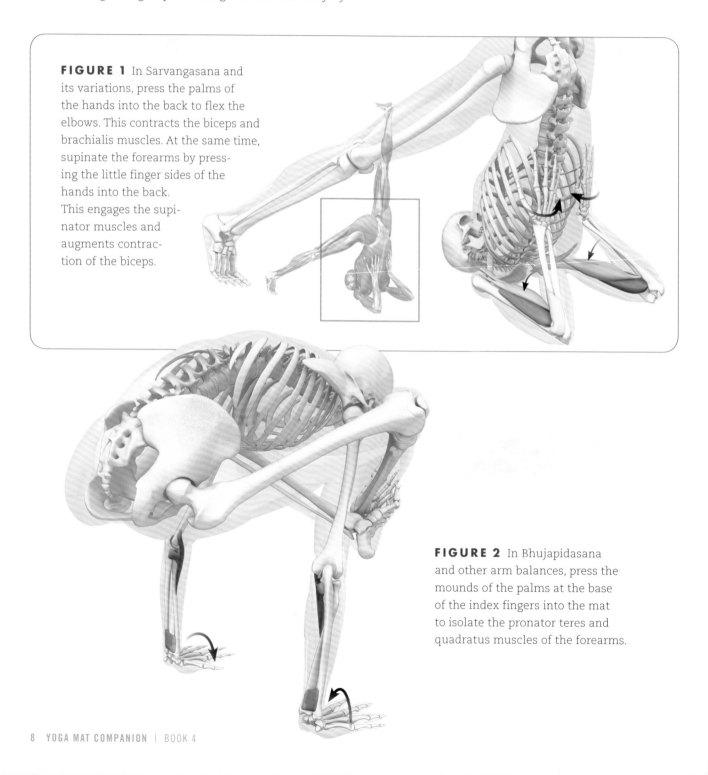

FIGURE 1 In Sarvangasana and its variations, press the palms of the hands into the back to flex the elbows. This contracts the biceps and brachialis muscles. At the same time, supinate the forearms by pressing the little finger sides of the hands into the back. This engages the supinator muscles and augments contraction of the biceps.

FIGURE 2 In Bhujapidasana and other arm balances, press the mounds of the palms at the base of the index fingers into the mat to isolate the pronator teres and quadratus muscles of the forearms.

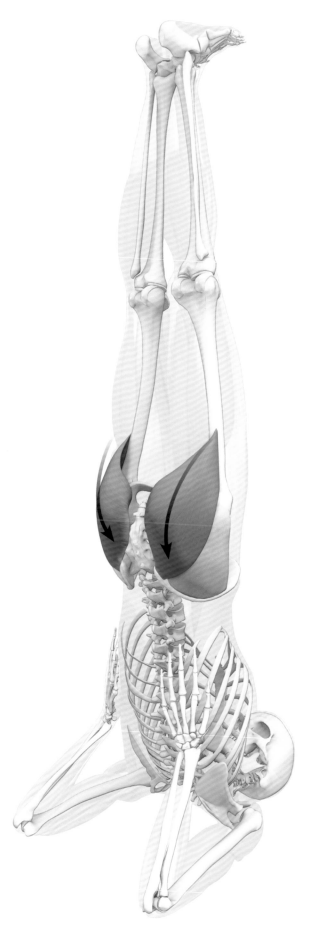

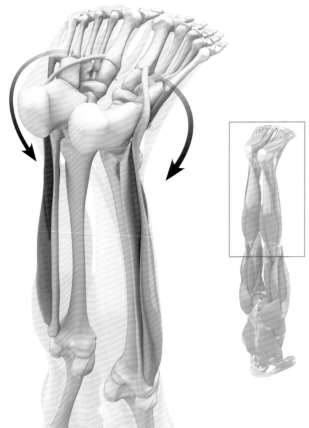

FIGURE 3 Tilt the sides of the feet outward, everting them in poses such as Headstand. This isolates the peroneus longus and brevis muscles at the sides of the lower legs.

◀ **FIGURE 4** The hips tend to flex forward in poses such as Sarvangasana. Correct this by engaging the buttocks muscles, including the gluteus maximus and medius. The cue for this action is to squeeze the buttocks.

KEY CONCEPT
KEY CO-ACTIVATIONS

Co-activation takes muscle isolation a step further. Here, two muscle groups engage simultaneously. Imagine two characters entering a scene together to move the plot along.

FIGURE 1 Activate the peroneus longus and brevis muscles to press the balls of the feet into the mat. Then, holding this action, engage the gluteus medius and tensor fascia lata (hip abductors) by attempting to drag the feet apart. The feet remain constrained on the mat, but contracting the gluteus medius and tensor fascia lata precipitates their secondary action—internal rotation of the hip. Use co-activation in this way to bring the kneecaps to face forward in Downward Facing Dog Pose.

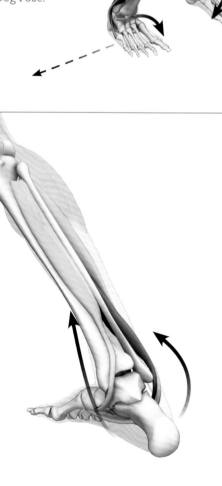

FIGURE 2 Steady the ankles in Downward Dog by first pressing the balls of the feet into the mat to activate the peroneus longus and brevis (the muscles that evert the midfoot). Hold this action and then spread the weight toward the outer edges of the feet to engage the tibialis posterior (the muscles that invert the midfoot). Feel how co-activating the peronei and tibialis posterior muscles secures the ankles.

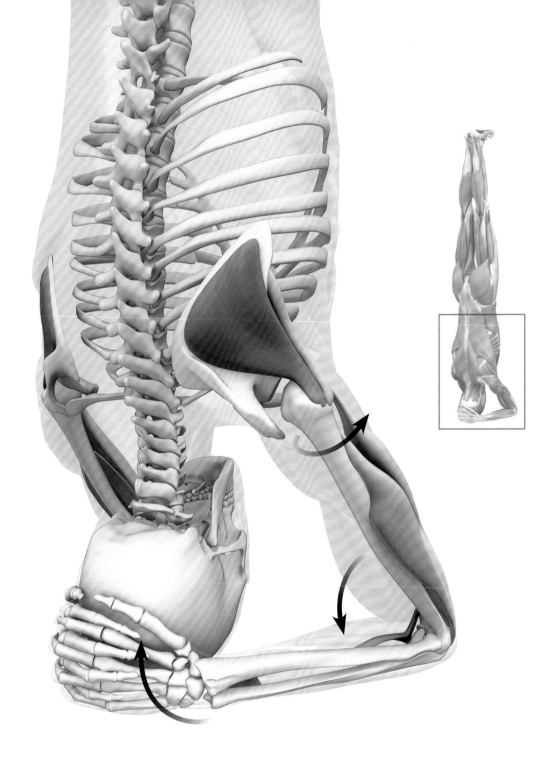

FIGURE 3 The shoulder girdle and arms establish the foundation of Sirsasana. Use co-activation of muscles and ligamentotaxis to secure this structure. Externally rotate the upper arm bones by contracting the infraspinatus and teres minor muscles of the rotator cuff. Then engage the triceps to press the edges of the forearms evenly into the mat. Finally, activate the pronators teres and quadratus to internally rotate the forearms and press the mounds of the palms (at the base of the index fingers) into the head. These combined actions produce a helical or "wringing" effect from the shoulder girdles to the hands and connect the foundation to the trunk. This stabilizes the inversion and protects the cervical spine.

KEY CONCEPT
CO-ACTIVATING SYNERGISTS

Synergist muscles can be used to refine and accentuate the actions of the agonists. Typically, muscles produce a primary action when they contract. They may also have secondary (and tertiary) actions based on the orientation of their fibers.

For example, the primary action of the adductor longus and brevis muscles is to adduct the hip joint. The orientation of their fibers also produces the secondary actions of flexing and externally rotating the hip. The tensor fascia lata, on the other side of this joint, has the primary action of abducting the hip and the secondary actions of flexing and internally rotating it. We can see that, although these muscles have primary actions that oppose each other, they also have a common secondary action—flexing the hip. Suppose we want to take advantage of this common function to synergize the prime mover of hip flexion, the psoas. We can do this by co-activating the adductors longus and brevis and the tensor fascia lata.

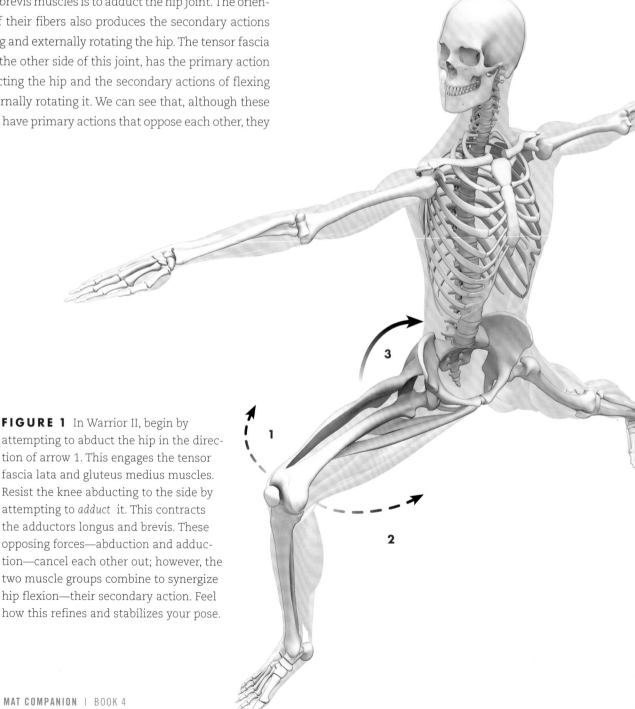

FIGURE 1 In Warrior II, begin by attempting to abduct the hip in the direction of arrow 1. This engages the tensor fascia lata and gluteus medius muscles. Resist the knee abducting to the side by attempting to *adduct* it. This contracts the adductors longus and brevis. These opposing forces—abduction and adduction—cancel each other out; however, the two muscle groups combine to synergize hip flexion—their secondary action. Feel how this refines and stabilizes your pose.

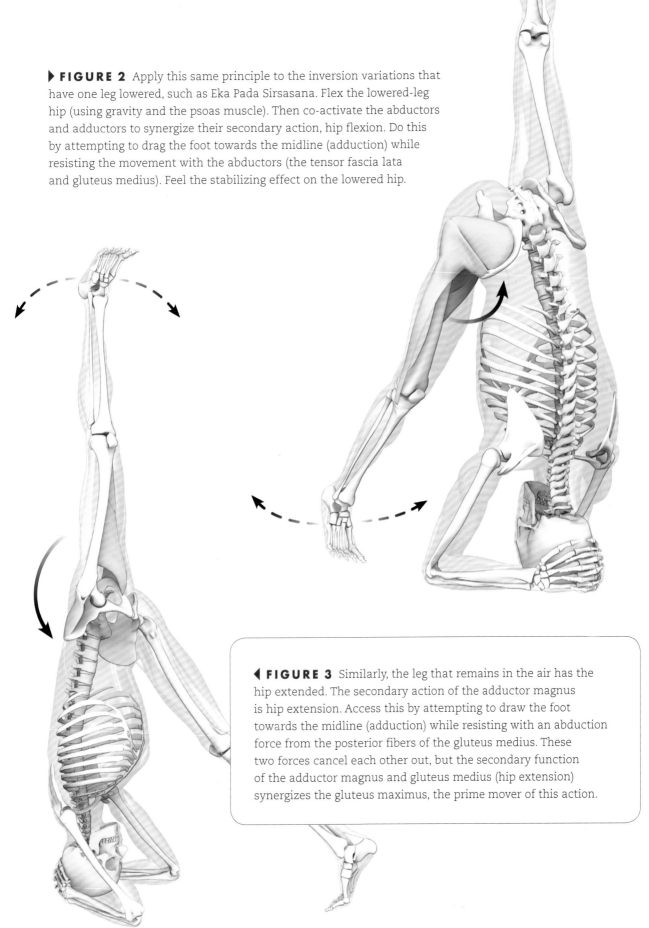

▶ **FIGURE 2** Apply this same principle to the inversion variations that have one leg lowered, such as Eka Pada Sirsasana. Flex the lowered-leg hip (using gravity and the psoas muscle). Then co-activate the abductors and adductors to synergize their secondary action, hip flexion. Do this by attempting to drag the foot towards the midline (adduction) while resisting the movement with the abductors (the tensor fascia lata and gluteus medius). Feel the stabilizing effect on the lowered hip.

◀ **FIGURE 3** Similarly, the leg that remains in the air has the hip extended. The secondary action of the adductor magnus is hip extension. Access this by attempting to draw the foot towards the midline (adduction) while resisting with an abduction force from the posterior fibers of the gluteus medius. These two forces cancel each other out, but the secondary function of the adductor magnus and gluteus medius (hip extension) synergizes the gluteus maximus, the prime mover of this action.

KEY CONCEPT
FACILITATED STRETCHES

Facilitated stretching works whether you understand its scientific reasoning or not. However, knowing the physiology behind each of these principles enables you to better integrate them, both mentally and physically. In the case of facilitated stretching, we intentionally contract the muscle we want to lengthen. This produces tension at the muscle-tendon junction, where a special nerve receptor is located—the Golgi tendon organ. This sensory receptor relays a message to the spinal cord about the state of tension in the muscle. The central nervous system acts as a mediator of this tension and prevents it from rising to dangerous levels. It does this by sending an inhibitory signal to the contractile elements of the muscle, producing an effect known as the relaxation response. In the period following this response, you can stretch the muscle and create a new "set length."

The set length of a muscle refers to your current level of flexibility in that region. Muscles lengthen or shorten to accommodate our habitual patterns of movement during activities of daily living. For example, someone who regularly rides a bicycle, like a triathlete in training, has their hips flexed a lot of the time. The same is true for people who sit for long periods at a desk. In these situations the set length of the hip flexors can become shortened. Stretching these muscles counterbalances this tendency.

Facilitated stretching is the most powerful method for increasing the set length of a muscle, and the regular practice of yoga maintains this increase. In addition, once you have achieved a new set length, even if you take some time away from stretching, the metaphorical "trail has been blazed," and it will be much easier to regain your previous flexibility.

Flexibility obtained from a regular practice makes activities of daily living easier. Your movement possibilities expand, and a sense of freedom is felt on all levels—physical, mental, and spiritual.

The main character in a facilitated stretch is the particular muscle that a practitioner is focusing on. Another way of looking at this is to consider that poses create a conflict between the muscles that contract and those that stretch—the agonists and the antagonists. When we activate a stretching muscle, as in facilitated stretching, we temporarily escalate that conflict. The central nervous system then negotiates a solution by causing the muscle to relax and lengthen into the stretch.

FIGURE 1 Spinal Cord Reflex Arc

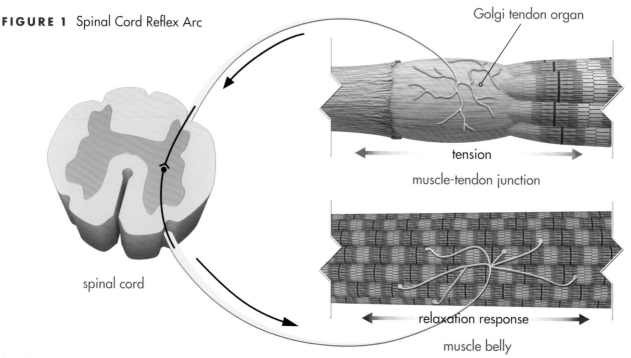

Golgi tendon organ

tension

muscle-tendon junction

spinal cord

relaxation response

muscle belly

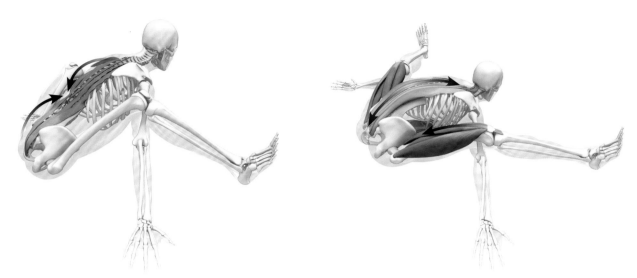

FIGURE 2 Use facilitated stretching to lengthen the back muscles in preparation for Tittibhasana. The best pose with which to do this is Kurmasana. Begin by placing the arms under the legs. Use the quadriceps to straighten the knees and press down onto the backs of the arms. Then attempt to arch the back. This contracts the erector spinae and quadratus lumborum—while they are stretching. In the process, tension at the muscle-tendon junction rises, stimulating the Golgi tendon organs located in this region. The Golgi tendon organs signal the central nervous system about the increased tension, and the central nervous system produces the relaxation response by inhibiting the muscle from contracting.

FIGURE 3 The next step is to take up the slack produced by the relaxation response to create a new set length for the muscle. Do this by relaxing the back and contracting the quadriceps to press down onto the arms. Co-activate the rectus abdominis to flex the trunk and go deeper into Tittibhasana.

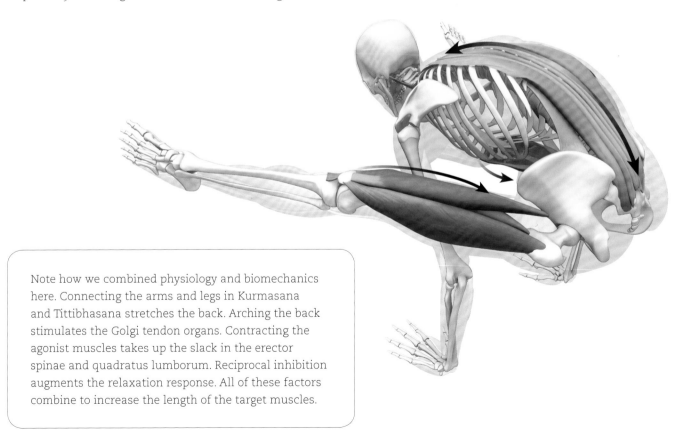

Note how we combined physiology and biomechanics here. Connecting the arms and legs in Kurmasana and Tittibhasana stretches the back. Arching the back stimulates the Golgi tendon organs. Contracting the agonist muscles takes up the slack in the erector spinae and quadratus lumborum. Reciprocal inhibition augments the relaxation response. All of these factors combine to increase the length of the target muscles.

KEY CONCEPT
BANDHAS

Bandhas, or "locks," are a form of co-activation that can be used to focus your mental gaze on a concise point in the pose. Facilitated stretching is an extension of co-activation that elevates this focus.

FIGURE 1 Use co-activation to create a bandha across the pelvis in the Eka Pada (or one-legged) variations of inversions. Do this by contracting the raised-leg side gluteus maximus to extend the hip. Combine this action with engaging the psoas on the lowered-leg side. The gluteus maximus retroverts its side of the pelvis, while the psoas anteverts the other side. These opposing forces combine to create a "wringing" effect across the sacroiliac joint, tightening its ligaments and stabilizing the pelvis. We illustrate this here with Eka Pada Sarvangasana.

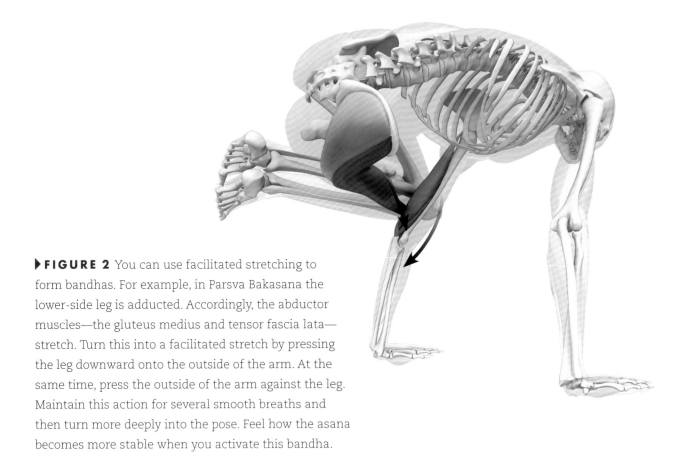

▶**FIGURE 2** You can use facilitated stretching to form bandhas. For example, in Parsva Bakasana the lower-side leg is adducted. Accordingly, the abductor muscles—the gluteus medius and tensor fascia lata—stretch. Turn this into a facilitated stretch by pressing the leg downward onto the outside of the arm. At the same time, press the outside of the arm against the leg. Maintain this action for several smooth breaths and then turn more deeply into the pose. Feel how the asana becomes more stable when you activate this bandha.

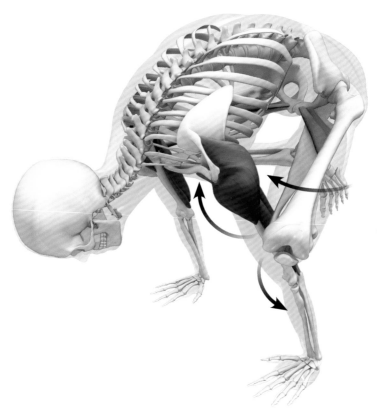

◀**FIGURE 3** Contract the adductor group to squeeze the inner thighs against the upper arms. At the same time, engage the lateral deltoids to press the arms outward against the thighs. Activate the triceps to extend the elbows. This links the upper and lower appendicular skeletons and creates a stabilizing bandha in Bakasana.

THE BANDHA YOGA CODEX

EACH YOGA POSTURE HAS ITS OWN UNIQUE FORM AND FUNCTION. MUSCLES THAT engage in one posture may be stretching in another. For this reason it helps to have a road map for navigating your way to the optimal pose. Better still is the ability to create your own road map. The Bandha Yoga Codex shows you how to do this.

There are five elements to every asana. These are the joint positions, the muscles that engage to produce these positions, the muscles that stretch, the breath, and the bandhas. Understanding the joint positions enables you to determine the muscles that produce the posture. Engage the prime movers to sculpt the pose, and polish it with the synergists. Once you know the prime movers, you can identify the muscles that are stretching. Apply physiological techniques to lengthen these muscles and create mobility to deepen the pose.

Then there is the breath. In virtually every posture we can benefit from expanding the chest. Combine the accessory muscles of breathing with the action of the diaphragm to increase the volume of the thorax. This improves oxygenation of the blood and removes energetic blockages in the subtle body.

The bandhas are the finishing touch. Co-activate the muscle groups that produce the joint positions and you will create bandhas throughout the body. Then connect these peripheral locks to the core bandhas. This produces stability in the pose and accentuates the sensory imprint of the asana on the mind.

The Bandha Yoga Codex is a five-step process that teaches how to identify these elements and decode any pose. This is your guide to creating a road map for combining science and yoga. I use Eka Pada Sarvangasana to illustrate the Codex on the following pages.

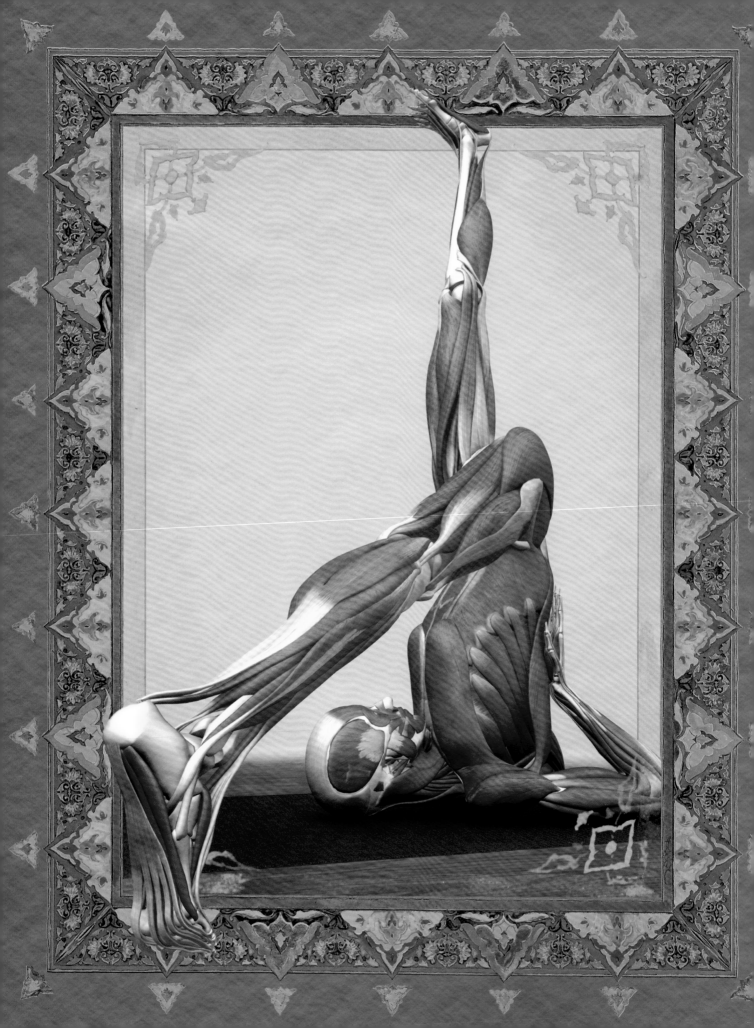

बन्ध योग

The Bandha Yoga Codex

— 1 —

Define the position of the joints in the pose.

— 2 —

Identify the prime mover muscles that act
on the joints to create the pose.
Contract these muscles to align and
stabilize the skeleton.

— 3 —

Identify the antagonist muscles
of the prime movers.
Stretch these muscles to create flexibility.

— 4 —

Expand the chest.

— 5 —

Create a Bandha.

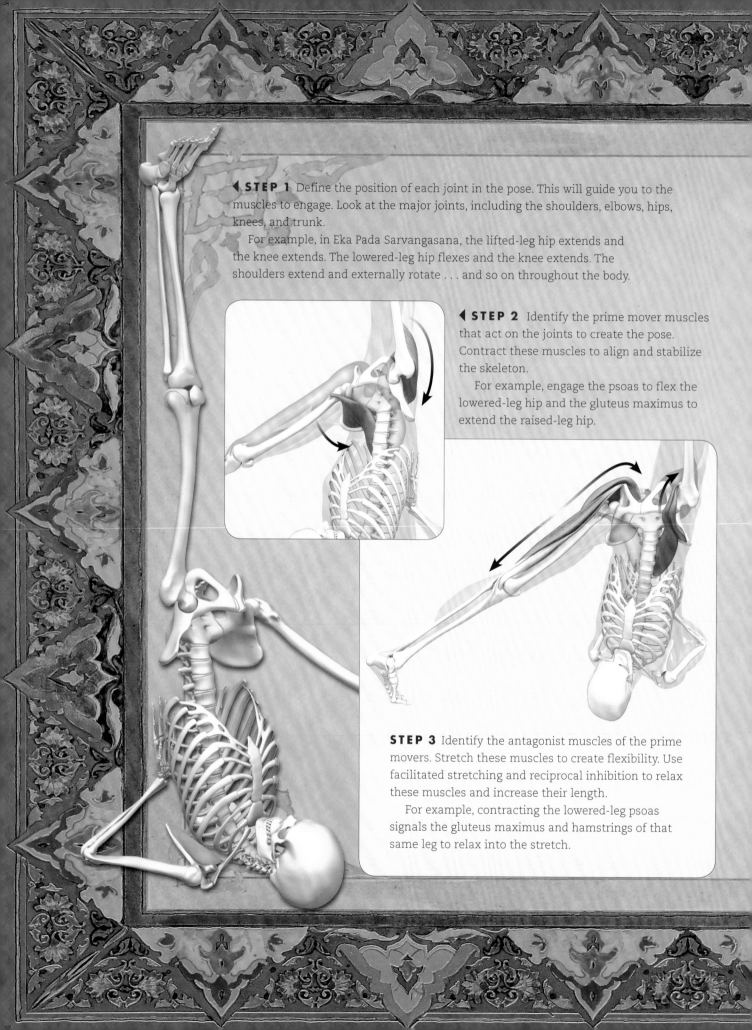

STEP 1 Define the position of each joint in the pose. This will guide you to the muscles to engage. Look at the major joints, including the shoulders, elbows, hips, knees, and trunk.

For example, in Eka Pada Sarvangasana, the lifted-leg hip extends and the knee extends. The lowered-leg hip flexes and the knee extends. The shoulders extend and externally rotate . . . and so on throughout the body.

STEP 2 Identify the prime mover muscles that act on the joints to create the pose. Contract these muscles to align and stabilize the skeleton.

For example, engage the psoas to flex the lowered-leg hip and the gluteus maximus to extend the raised-leg hip.

STEP 3 Identify the antagonist muscles of the prime movers. Stretch these muscles to create flexibility. Use facilitated stretching and reciprocal inhibition to relax these muscles and increase their length.

For example, contracting the lowered-leg psoas signals the gluteus maximus and hamstrings of that same leg to relax into the stretch.

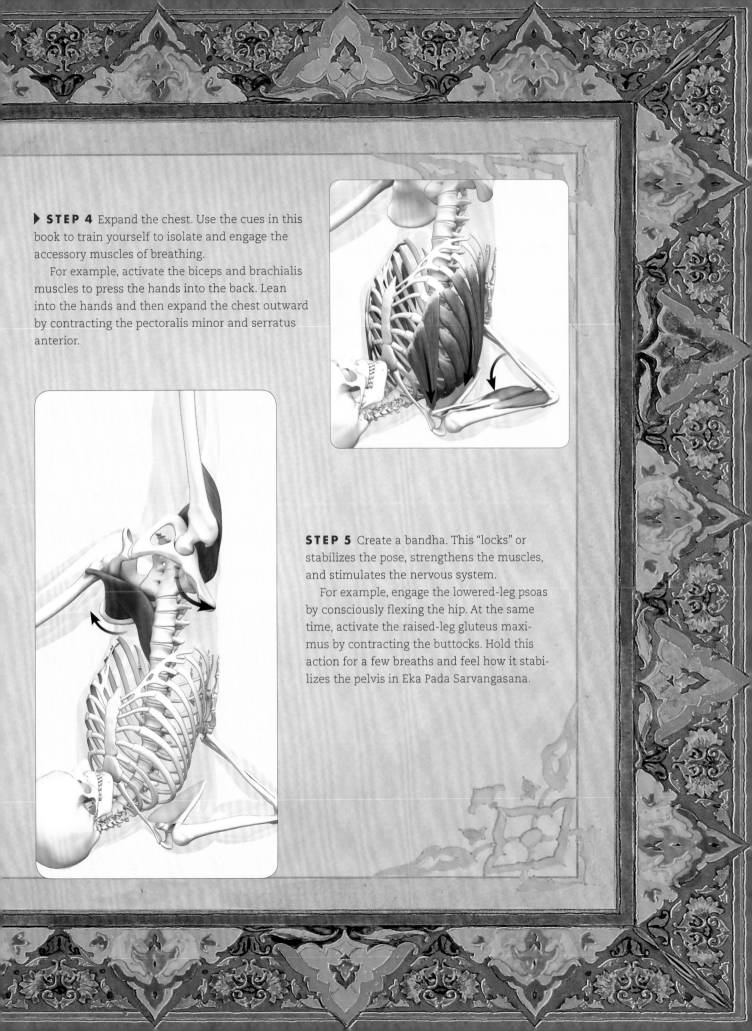

▶ **STEP 4** Expand the chest. Use the cues in this book to train yourself to isolate and engage the accessory muscles of breathing.

For example, activate the biceps and brachialis muscles to press the hands into the back. Lean into the hands and then expand the chest outward by contracting the pectoralis minor and serratus anterior.

STEP 5 Create a bandha. This "locks" or stabilizes the pose, strengthens the muscles, and stimulates the nervous system.

For example, engage the lowered-leg psoas by consciously flexing the hip. At the same time, activate the raised-leg gluteus maximus by contracting the buttocks. Hold this action for a few breaths and feel how it stabilizes the pelvis in Eka Pada Sarvangasana.

ARM
BALANCES

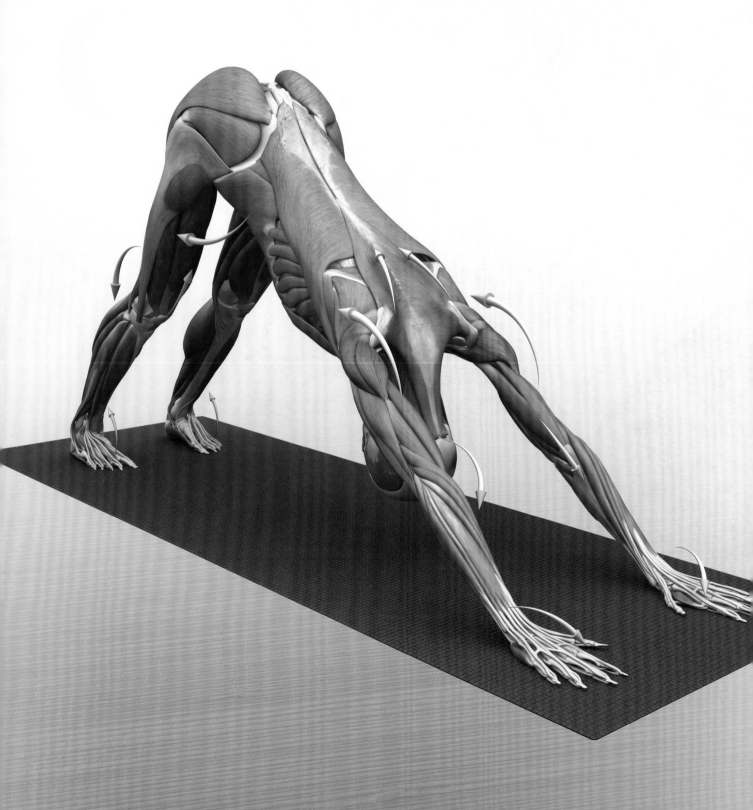

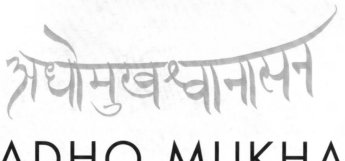

ADHO MUKHA SVANASANA
DOWNWARD FACING DOG POSE

ADHO MUKHA SVANASANA IS BOTH AN INVERSION AND AN ARM BALANCE. IT IS THE resting point in the Vinyasa sequence and serves as a barometer for the stretch at the backs of the legs as well as the shoulders. Flexing the hips and straightening the knees focuses the stretch on the hamstrings. You can dorsiflex the feet to emphasize the stretch of the gastrocnemius (which crosses the backs of the knees) and soleus (which crosses the ankles with the gastrocnemius). Straightening the arms to press the body back toward the legs indirectly deepens the stretch. Address these basic movements first. From there you can focus on the nuances of Dog Pose, remembering that many of the most profound experiences of yoga take place with small, concentrated, and subtle movements. For example, pronating the forearms while externally rotating the shoulders creates a "coiling" helical effect up and down the lengths of the arms; this tightens the elbow ligaments and stabilizes the pose. Another subplot in the story involves opening the wings of the iliac bones to allow the sacrum to tilt forward. Do this by attempting to "scrub" the feet outward on the mat. This engages the abductor muscles in a closed chain fashion, moving their origins on the iliac crest. Engage the buttocks by attempting to scrub the feet away from the hands. Pronate the ankles by pressing the weight into the balls of the feet. Then lift the arches to spread the weight to the outer edges. This balance of eversion and inversion at the ankles stabilizes the pose from its foundation. You can use any or all of these nuances as you walk through and deepen the asana.

BASIC JOINT POSITIONS

- The hips flex.
- The knees extend.
- The shoulders flex and externally rotate.
- The elbows extend.
- The forearms pronate.
- The wrists extend.
- The ankles dorsiflex.
- The lumbar spine extends.
- The cervical spine flexes.

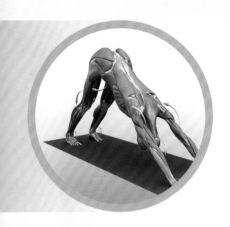

Adho Mukha Svanasana
Preparation

Adho Mukha Svanasana is practiced as a free-standing posture or as part of a Vinyasa sequence. If you're using it in Vinyasa, then for the first few rounds, simply take the basic shape of the pose by flexing the hips and straightening the knees and elbows. This prepares the major muscle groups that are stretching. Once you are warmed up, begin adding synergist muscles to refine the pose, as described in the steps that follow.

For the free-standing version, begin on all four. Get a feel for pressing the palms into the mat. Spread the fingers evenly apart and rotate the shoulders outward. Turn the toes under to place the weight onto the mounds of the feet. Lift the knees and flex the trunk toward the thighs. Activate the triceps to straighten the arms. Then, keeping the trunk flexed, straighten the knees to come up into the pose. Ease out of Downward Facing Dog by bending the knees and coming back to the floor. Rest in Child's Pose.

You can use the chair stretch illustrated below to lengthen the shoulder extensor muscles. Turn this into a facilitated stretch by pressing the elbows onto the seat of the chair for several breaths. Then take up the slack produced by the relaxation response.

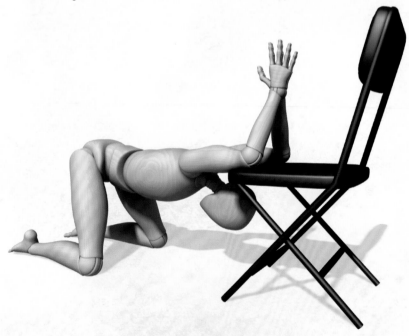

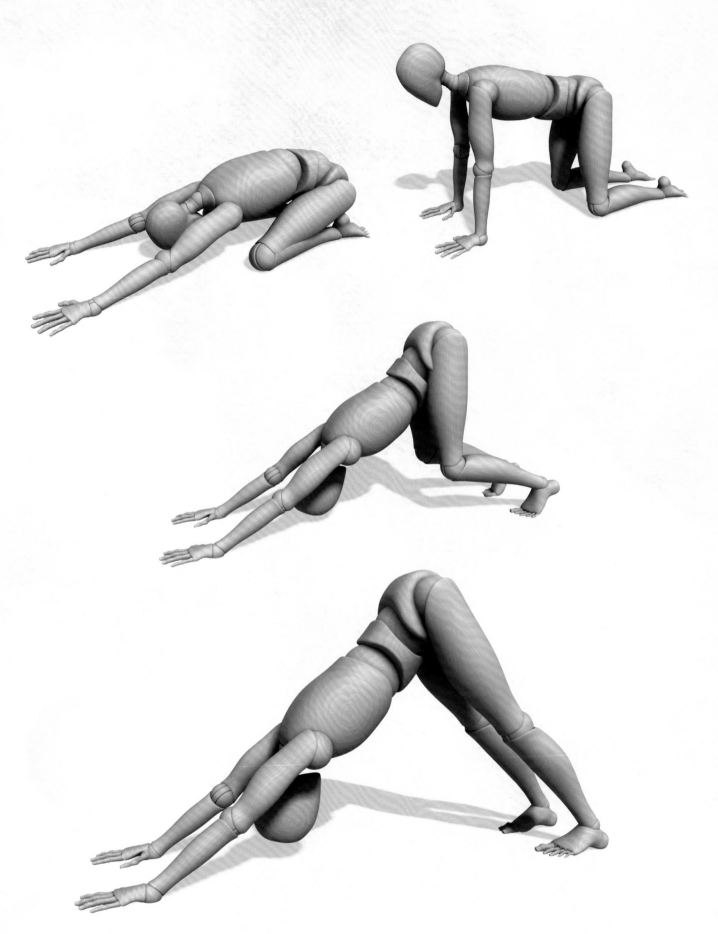

ADHO MUKHA SVANASANA—DOWNWARD FACING DOG POSE **29**

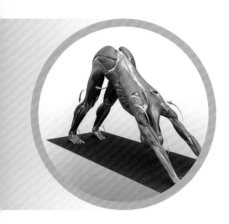

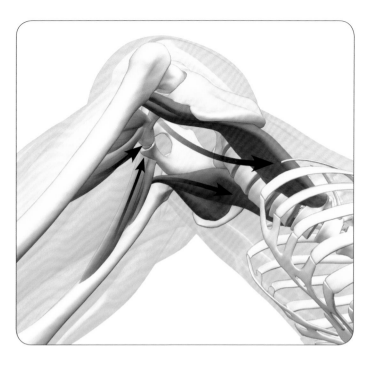

STEP 1 Flex the hips by contracting the psoas muscle and its synergists, including the adductors longus and brevis and the pectineus. A cue for engaging these muscles is to attempt to drag the feet towards one another. Bend the knees at first. This releases the pull of the hamstrings on the ischial tuberosities and allows the pelvis to tilt forward when the psoas contracts. Note the origin of the psoas major on the lumbar spine. Engaging this muscle also draws the lumbar spine forward, slightly arching the lower back. This is a desired form for Dog Pose. Activating the psoas produces reciprocal inhibition of the gluteus maximus (a hip extensor).

STEP 2 Several muscles synergize the actions of the psoas. The pectineus and adductors longus and brevis flex the hips and tilt the pelvis forward. The sartorius and rectus femoris also flex the hips, since they cross the joint on their way to the knee. Note the origins of these muscles on the anterior superior iliac spine (ASIS) and the anterior inferior iliac spine (AIIS). Activating them draws the pelvis forward. A cue for contracting the rectus femoris is to lift the kneecap (where the muscle inserts). The sartorius is more difficult to isolate, but it will engage when you flex the hip, especially if you externally rotate the femur. The gluteus minimus crosses the hip on the outside of the ilium. Its action varies depending on whether the hip is flexing, neutral, or extending. The hips flex in Dog Pose, at which time the gluteus minimus also acts as a flexor. The gluteus minimus is a small muscle that lies deep to the other gluteals, making it difficult to contract at will; use visualization to engage it.

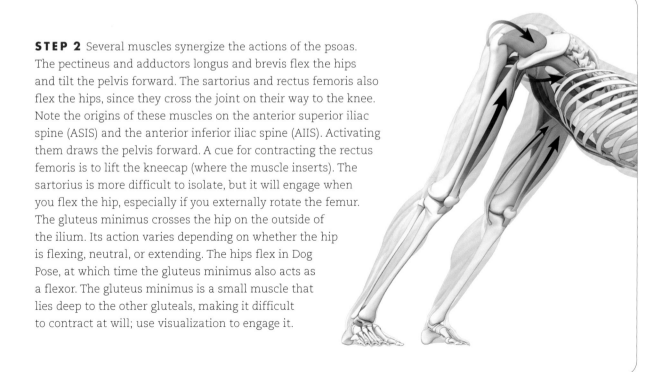

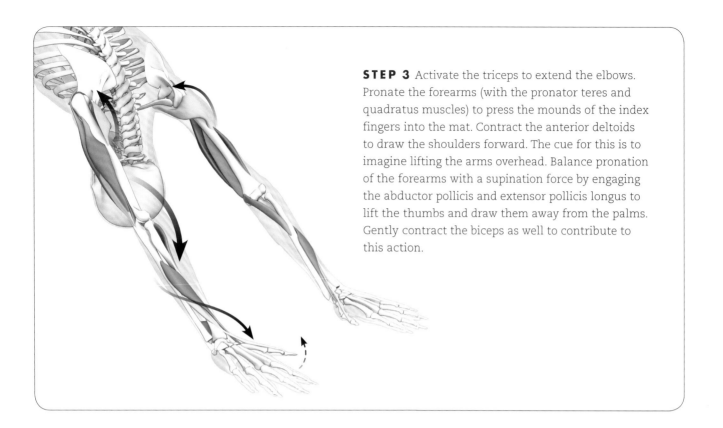

STEP 3 Activate the triceps to extend the elbows. Pronate the forearms (with the pronator teres and quadratus muscles) to press the mounds of the index fingers into the mat. Contract the anterior deltoids to draw the shoulders forward. The cue for this is to imagine lifting the arms overhead. Balance pronation of the forearms with a supination force by engaging the abductor pollicis and extensor pollicis longus to lift the thumbs and draw them away from the palms. Gently contract the biceps as well to contribute to this action.

STEP 4 Engage the quadriceps to extend the knees. Activate the gluteus medius and tensor fascia lata to draw the iliac bones slightly apart (through closed chain contraction) and internally rotate the thighs. A cue for this is to fix the feet on the mat and then attempt to scrub them away from each other. Because the feet won't move, the force of this contraction is transmuted to internal rotation, creating a "coiling" line of force down the legs.

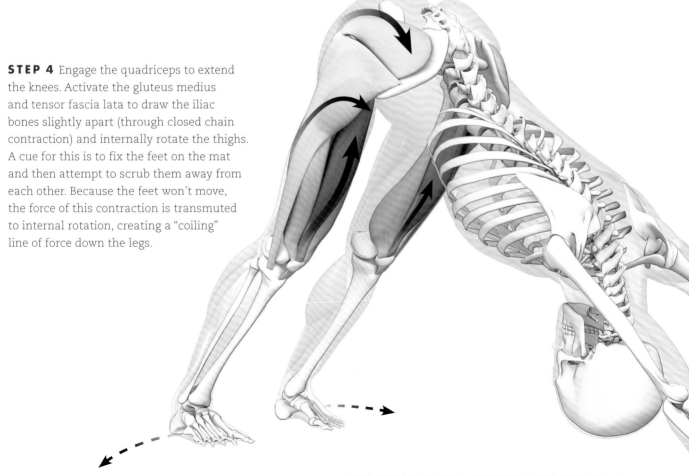

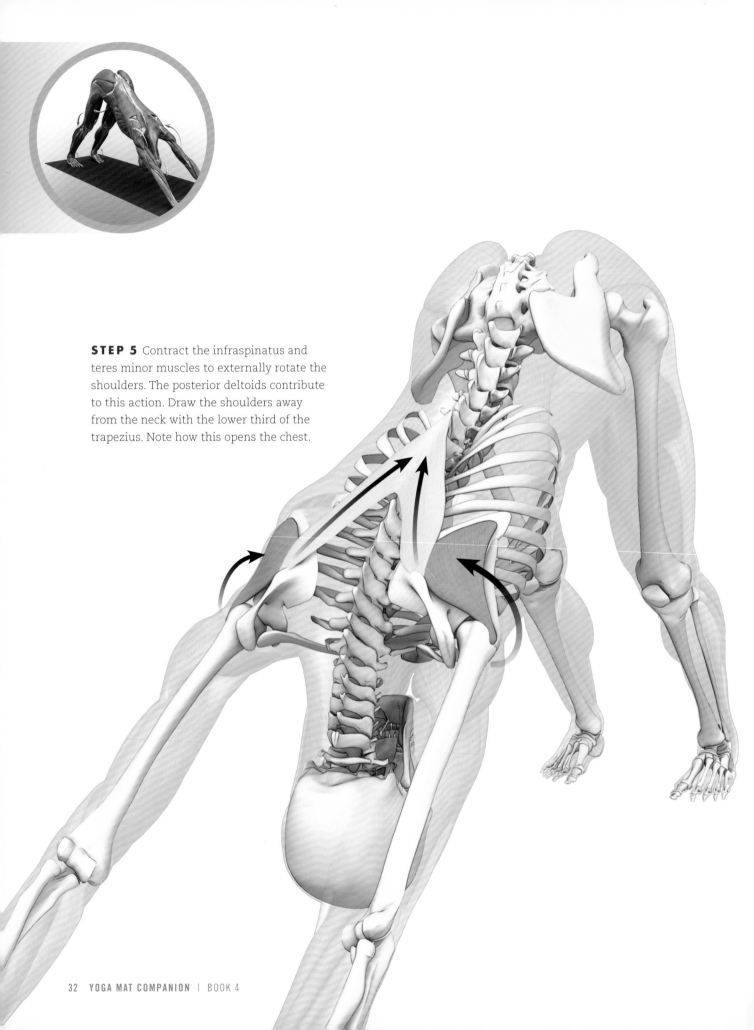

STEP 5 Contract the infraspinatus and teres minor muscles to externally rotate the shoulders. The posterior deltoids contribute to this action. Draw the shoulders away from the neck with the lower third of the trapezius. Note how this opens the chest.

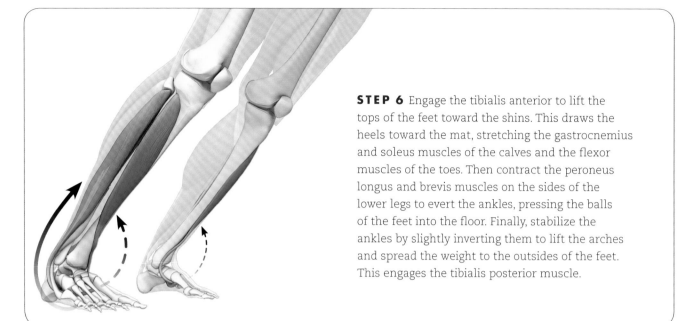

STEP 6 Engage the tibialis anterior to lift the tops of the feet toward the shins. This draws the heels toward the mat, stretching the gastrocnemius and soleus muscles of the calves and the flexor muscles of the toes. Then contract the peroneus longus and brevis muscles on the sides of the lower legs to evert the ankles, pressing the balls of the feet into the floor. Finally, stabilize the ankles by slightly inverting them to lift the arches and spread the weight to the outsides of the feet. This engages the tibialis posterior muscle.

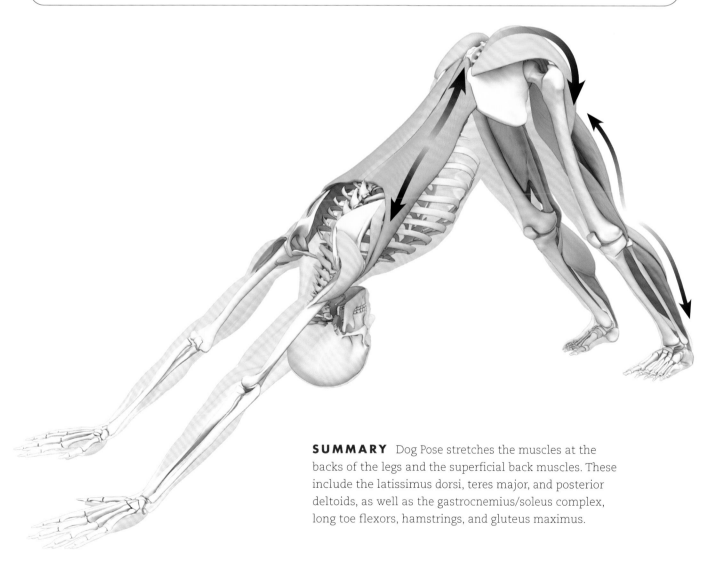

SUMMARY Dog Pose stretches the muscles at the backs of the legs and the superficial back muscles. These include the latissimus dorsi, teres major, and posterior deltoids, as well as the gastrocnemius/soleus complex, long toe flexors, hamstrings, and gluteus maximus.

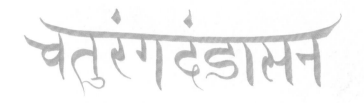

CHATURANGA DANDASANA

FOUR-LIMBED STAFF POSE

CHATURANGA DANDASANA CAN BE PRACTICED AS A FREE-STANDING POSE OR AS part of the Vinyasa sequence, typically coming after Uttanasana by jumping or stepping back. Anticipate in your mind the muscles that you will engage to lower the body into the pose, including the chest and shoulder muscles, as the weight is taken into the arms. There is a tendency for the pelvis to sag downward in Chaturanga. Plan for this and counter it by activating the trunk flexors. Similarly, you can sequentially contract various muscle groups to press up into the pose from the floor. For example, engage the pectoralis major, serratus anterior, and triceps muscles to lift the chest. Straighten the knees by contracting the quadriceps. Then activate the psoas and rectus abdominis to lift the pelvis. These actions produce an effect that is like scaffolding or the spans of a suspension bridge. Stabilize this structure by creating a counterforce between the muscles of the ankles and feet pushing the body forward and the core muscles of the shoulders pressing the body back. These combined actions create a peripheral lock (or bandha) that can be used to recruit the muscles of the pelvic diaphragm and accentuate mula bandha. This is an example of co-activation.

BASIC JOINT POSITIONS

- The elbows flex.
- The forearms pronate.
- The wrists extend.
- The shoulders externally rotate.
- The knees extend.

- The ankles dorsiflex.
- The toes extend.
- The hips are neutral.
- The spine is neutral.

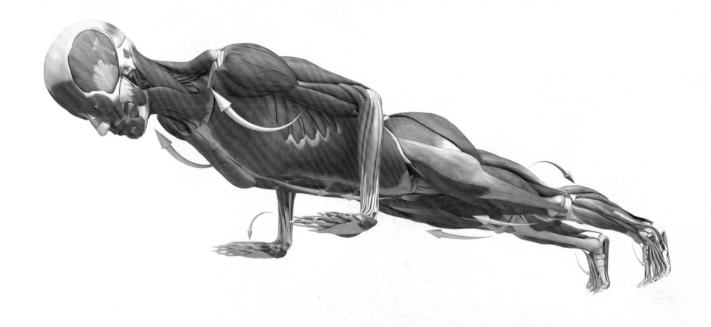

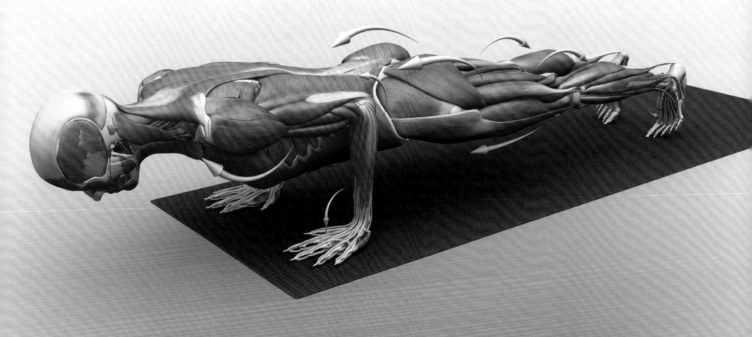

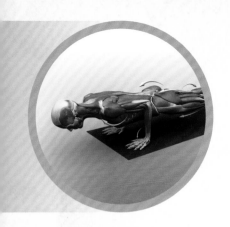

Chaturanga Dandasana
Preparation

The preparation shows how to enter Chaturanga from the floor. You can also enter from a high push-up position, for example, from the Sun Salutation sequence.

Place the hands on the floor and press forward, as if trying to straighten the elbows. This lifts the chest while the pelvis and thighs remain on the mat. Then engage the quadriceps to straighten the knees. Contract the hip and trunk flexors (the psoas and abdominals) to lift the pelvis like a suspension bridge. Keep the abdominals engaged for support. Finally, activate the buttocks to balance the force of the contracting hip flexors and to stabilize the pelvis in a neutral position.

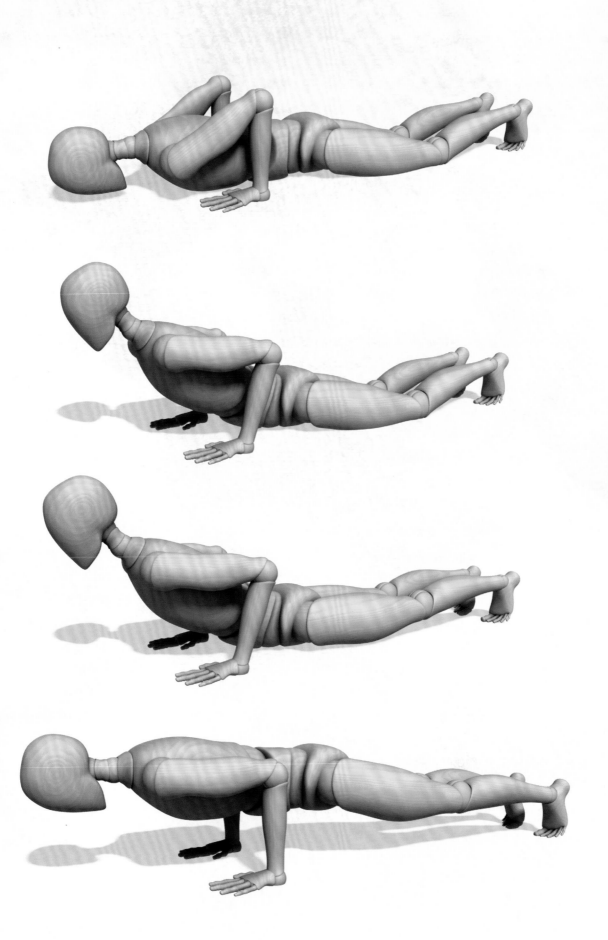

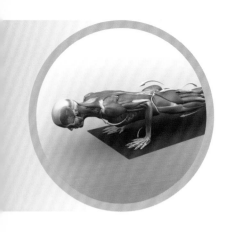

STEP 1 Press the mounds at the base of the index fingers into the mat by engaging the pronator teres and quadratus muscles to pronate the forearms. This activates the arches of the palms. Contract the triceps to attempt to straighten the elbows and lift the chest from the floor. Then draw the shoulder blades toward the midline of the spine and away from the neck using the rhomboids and lower third of the trapezius, respectively.

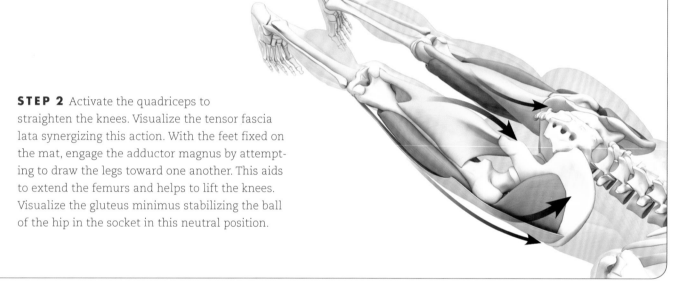

STEP 2 Activate the quadriceps to straighten the knees. Visualize the tensor fascia lata synergizing this action. With the feet fixed on the mat, engage the adductor magnus by attempting to draw the legs toward one another. This aids to extend the femurs and helps to lift the knees. Visualize the gluteus minimus stabilizing the ball of the hip in the socket in this neutral position.

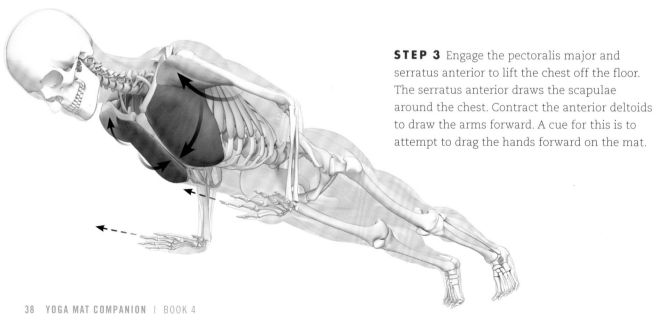

STEP 3 Engage the pectoralis major and serratus anterior to lift the chest off the floor. The serratus anterior draws the scapulae around the chest. Contract the anterior deltoids to draw the arms forward. A cue for this is to attempt to drag the hands forward on the mat.

STEP 4 Lifting the knees and the chest off the floor creates a concave curve throughout the body, with the apex at the pelvis. Turn this curve into a straight line by activating the psoas and its synergists; this flexes the hips and lifts them off the floor. At the same time, grip the rectus abdominis to stabilize the pelvis in the air. Remember that contracting the abdominal muscles raises intra-abdominal pressure, making it harder for the diaphragm to flatten and draw air into the lungs. Counter this by breathing deeply.

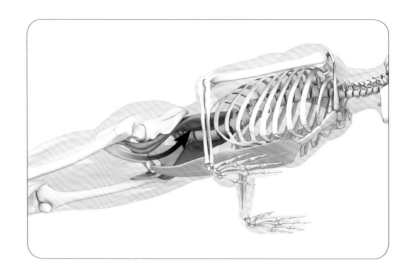

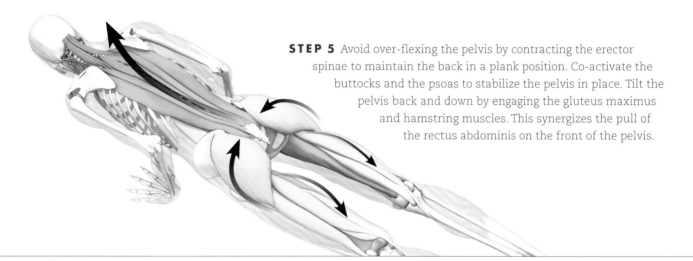

STEP 5 Avoid over-flexing the pelvis by contracting the erector spinae to maintain the back in a plank position. Co-activate the buttocks and the psoas to stabilize the pelvis in place. Tilt the pelvis back and down by engaging the gluteus maximus and hamstring muscles. This synergizes the pull of the rectus abdominis on the front of the pelvis.

STEP 6 Attempt to scrub the mat forward with the hands. This activates the biceps and brachialis muscles and stabilizes the elbows. The anterior deltoids synergize this action, as described in Step 3. Then attempt to press the toes backwards on the mat, as if coming out of a starting block. This shifts the weight towards the hands, while the hands resist and press the weight backwards towards the feet. In this way, co-activation of the elbow and ankle flexors combines with the actions of the other muscles described to support the "suspension bridge" across the front of the body.

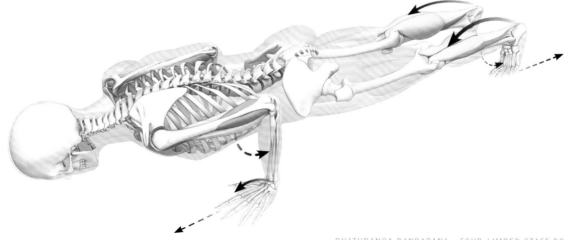

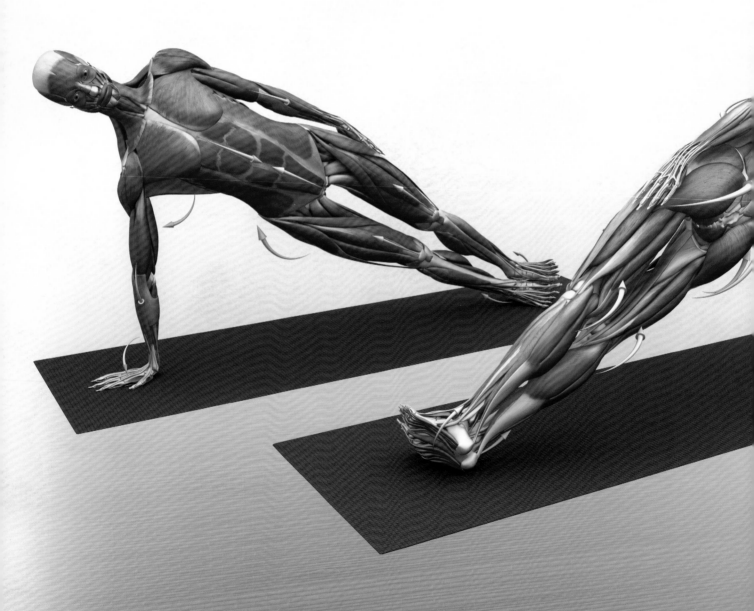

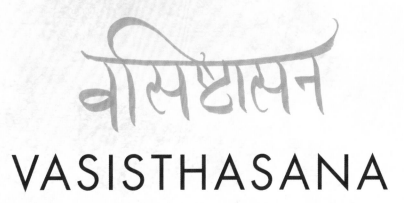

VASISTHASANA

SAGE POSE

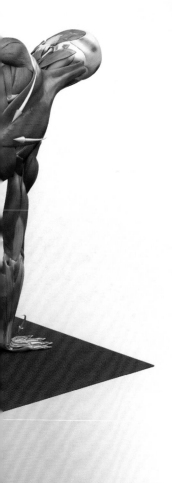

VASISTHASANA HAS THREE MAIN FOCI OR STORIES: THE ARM THAT IS HOLDING the body up, the lower-side leg, and the pelvis. Each interacts with the other to create balance. The hand connects with the shoulder via the wrist, elbow, and upper arm. It ultimately connects with the thorax through contraction of the serratus anterior. This muscle wraps around the chest from the scapula and helps stabilize the shoulder blade against the chest wall. In addition to stabilizing the shoulder, the serratus anterior can be used to expand the ribcage, making it an accessory muscle of breathing. Use Vasisthasana to become aware of how this important muscle feels when it contracts. Then apply this awareness to expand the chest during inhalation in other asanas. This is an example of awakening muscles with yoga.

On the lower-side leg, the peroneus longus and brevis evert the foot at the ankle. Tilting the ankle into eversion brings the outer edge of the foot firmly into contact with the floor, stabilizing the leg. Although the lower-side arm and leg lift the body, it would sag considerably if the muscles at the side of the pelvis did not engage. Because the foot is fixed on the mat, activating the muscles that abduct the leg creates a force that lifts the pelvis. This is an example of closed chain contraction, wherein the insertion of the muscle remains fixed and the origin moves (in this case, the pelvis lifts).

Subplots of the pose include pressing the upper-side hand against the side of the body and attempting to drag it backwards. This engages the latissimus dorsi in a closed chain fashion, levering the chest open. Activate the quadriceps to lift the kneecaps and straighten the legs. Contract the adductor muscles to squeeze the knees together. Firm the abdomen to obtain stability in the pose.

BASIC JOINT POSITIONS

- The lower-side shoulder abducts and externally rotates.
- The upper-side shoulder adducts and externally rotates.
- The elbows extend.
- The forearms pronate.
- The knees extend.
- The lower-side hip abducts.
- The upper-side hip adducts.
- The ankles dorsiflex.
- The feet evert.
- The spine is neutral.

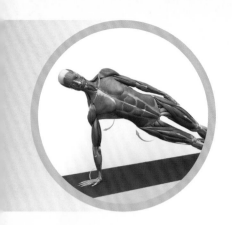

Vasisthasana Preparation

Begin in a push-up position. This activates some of the same muscles that you will use for Vasisthasana. Extend the elbows and draw the scapulae away from the midline of the back. Engage the abdomen. When you have enough strength to hold this position, then progress to one arm by lifting the other arm up and bringing the upper foot to the floor in front of the body, as shown.

The pelvis will sag at first. Get a feeling for lifting it by activating the abductor muscles on the sides of the hips and the lower-side abdominals. To gain awareness of these muscles, lift the pelvis up and down a few times, pressing the side of the foot into the floor.

When you feel balanced, bring the upper leg onto the bottom leg and squeeze the thighs together. Engage the buttocks and extend the back to open the chest. You can raise the upper hand toward the ceiling or place it on the thigh; experience the different effects of each. For example, balance is easier with the hand on the thigh because the center of gravity is lower. Breathe. Ease out of the pose by reversing the process.

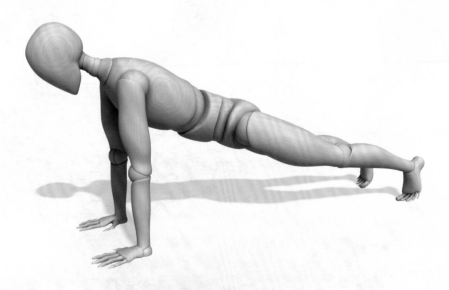

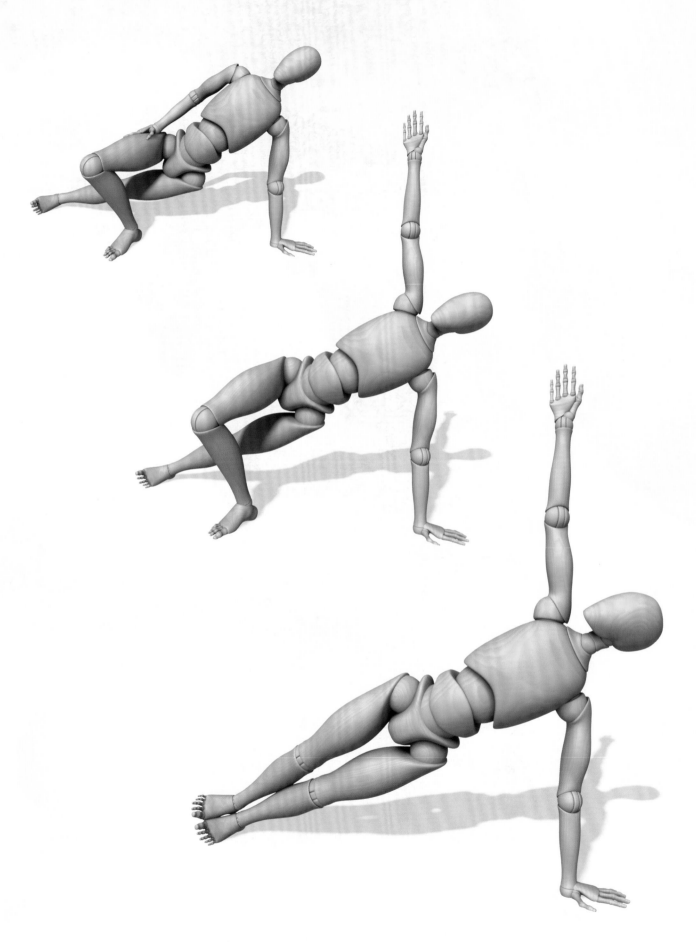

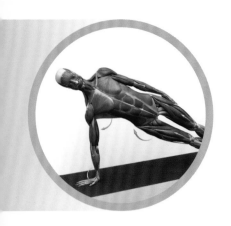

STEP 1 Place the hand on the floor, pronating the forearm and spreading the weight across the palm. Grip the fingers to activate the palmar arch. The pronators teres and quadratus turn the hand downward and press the inner surface of the hand into the floor. Flex the wrist by pressing the mounds at the base of the fingers into the mat to engage the flexors carpi radialis and ulnaris and stabilize the wrist. Contract the triceps to extend the elbow. The long head of this muscle has its origin on the scapula; consequently, engaging it contributes stability to the shoulder. If your elbow hyperextends, then attempt to bend it by co-contracting the biceps; this aligns the upper and lower arm bones. Activate the serratus anterior to abduct the scapula away from the midline by pressing down from the shoulder through the hand. Maintain the arm perpendicular to the floor, so that the force of gravity (the mechanical axis) aligns with the bones' long anatomical axes.

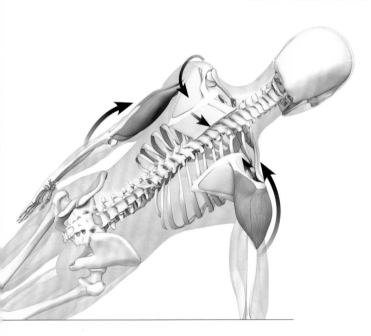

◀ **STEP 2** Activate the lateral deltoid to lift the torso and abduct the shoulder. The supraspinatus of the rotator cuff initiates this action and helps stabilize the head of the humerus in the socket. Slightly externally rotate the shoulder and elbow with the infraspinatus, teres minor, and posterior portion of the deltoid. Draw the upper-side scapula toward the midline by engaging the rhomboids on that side. This expands the chest forward. Engage the triceps of the upper-side arm to straighten the elbow.

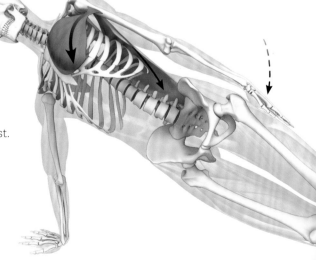

▶ **STEP 3** Press the hand into the side of the thigh (adduction) by engaging the pectoralis and teres major muscles. This also lifts the chest. To get a sense of what it's like to have the pectoralis major contract, before going into the pose, press the hand against your side. Feel the muscle engage with your other hand by placing it on your chest.

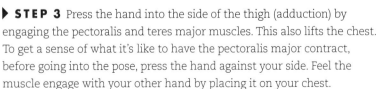

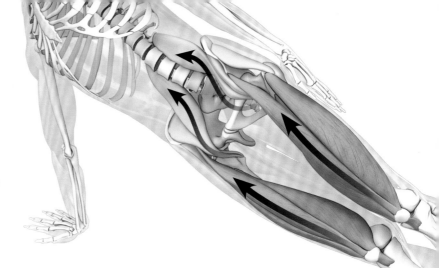

▶ **STEP 4** Engage the quadriceps to extend the knees. Visualize the gluteus minimus contracting to stabilize the ball of the hip in the socket. Activate the psoas to counterbalance the extension force of the gluteus maximus and prevent swayback.

STEP 5 Press the side of the foot into the floor, everting it and dorsiflexing the ankle so that the foot forms a right angle with the tibia. The peroneus longus and brevis muscles evert the foot. The extensor digitorum longus synergizes this and draws the toes up. Activate the tibialis anterior on the front of the lower leg to dorsiflex the foot. Contract the gluteus medius and tensor fascia lata to lift the pelvis at the hip by pressing the side of the foot into the floor. The force of this action is transmitted to moving the trunk upward and stabilizing it there.

▶ **STEP 6** Engage the back extensors, including the erector spinae and quadratus lumborum. The lower side engages relatively more forcefully to lift the trunk and prevent sagging. Contract the gluteus maximus to extend the hips and stabilize the pelvis. The cue for this is to tuck the tailbone under.

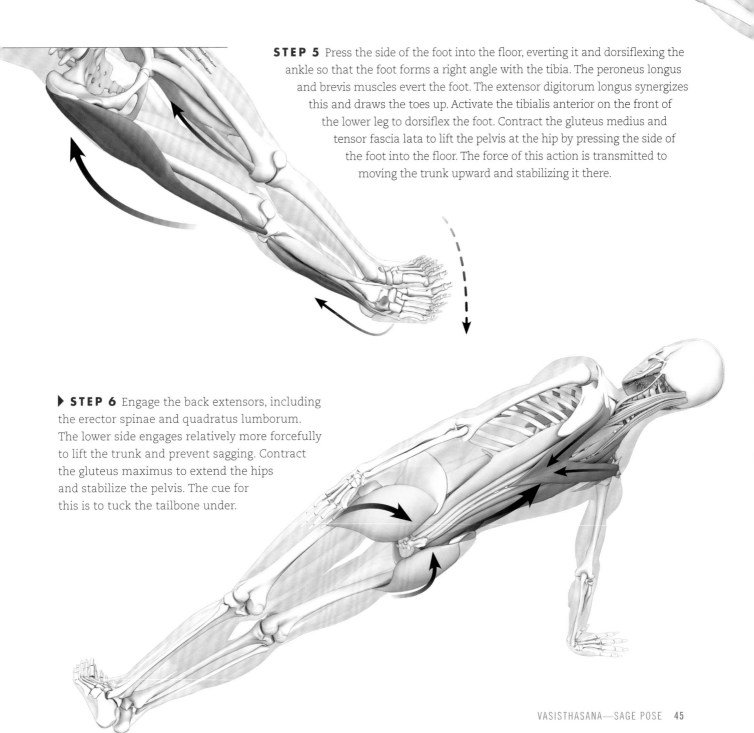

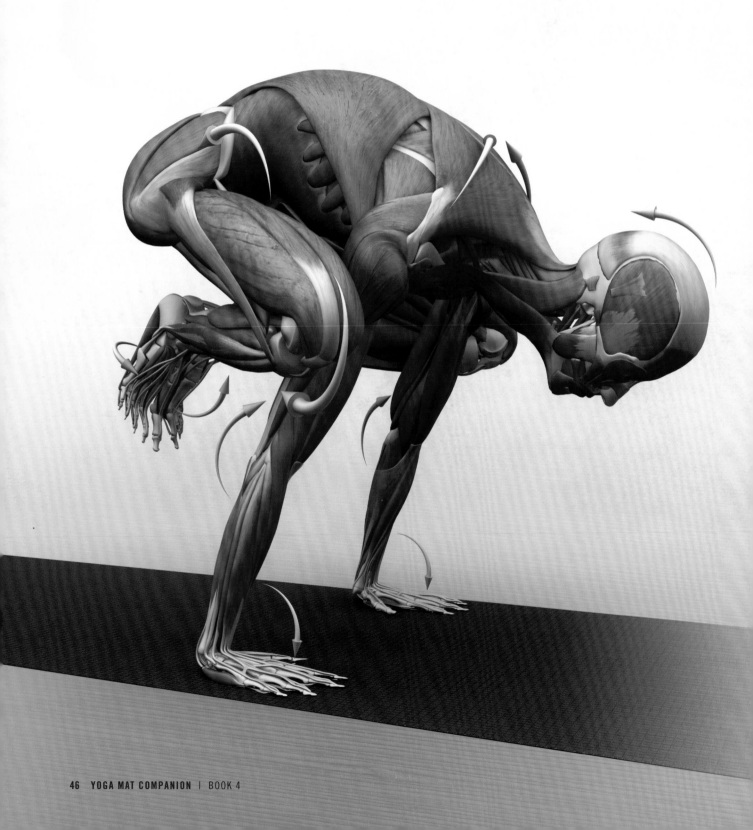

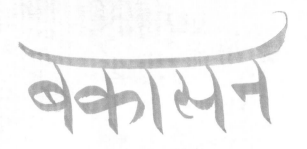

BAKASANA

CRANE POSE

ALIGNMENT IS AS IMPORTANT AS STRENGTH IN THIS AND OTHER ARM BALANCES. Engaging the correct muscles provides the necessary force required for stability. Bakasana connects the upper and lower extremities at the inner thighs and upper arms. The powerful muscles of the inner legs—the adductors—are at an optimal length to generate force with the least amount of effort. In Bakasana, the legs use these muscles to grip the arms and create a focus for balance. Firmly extend the elbows to lift the body, placing the center of gravity directly down through the hands. Activate the abdominals to flex and lift the trunk upwards. Flex the hips and knees to draw the feet up, and evert the ankles to open the soles of the feet as the final element of the pose.

BASIC JOINT POSITIONS

- The hips flex and adduct.
- The knees flex.
- The ankles dorsiflex.
- The feet evert.
- The toes extend.
- The trunk flexes.

- The shoulders flex, adduct, and externally rotate.
- The elbows extend.
- The forearms pronate.
- The wrists extend.
- The cervical spine extends.

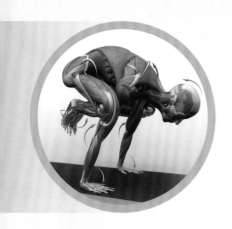

Bakasana Preparation

Stand on a block. Bend down and squeeze the inner knees against the outer arms to feel the adductor muscles contract. Engage the abdominals and hip flexors to begin to lift up and push off the block with the feet. Activate the muscles at the front of the chest, as well as the abdominals, as you squeeze the knees against the arms. This helps to maintain the pose. Then carefully rock backward onto the toes to come out. You may want to put a bolster or blanket in front of you as a cushion (in case of a "face plant").

You can use forward bends such as Uttanasana to prepare the lower back muscles and gluteals for the stretch in Bakasana.

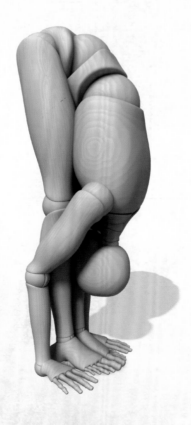

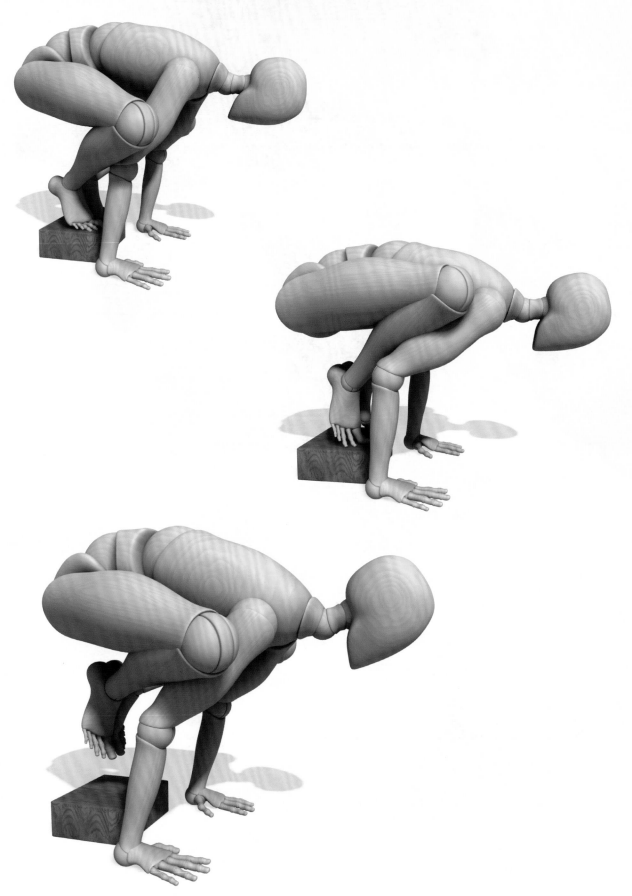

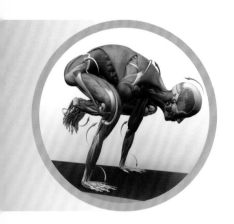

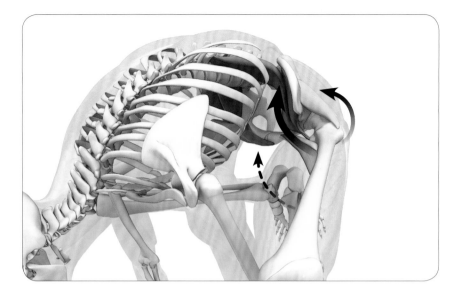

STEP 1 Contract the psoas, pectineus, and adductors longus and brevis at the front of the pelvis to flex the hips. The gluteus minimus on the side of the pelvis also becomes a hip flexor in this position, aiding to draw the thighs up onto the sides of the arms. Engage the rectus abdominis to flex the lower trunk and draw the pubic symphysis at the front of the pelvis forward.

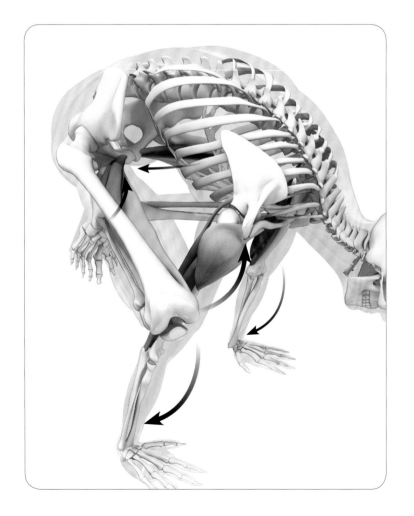

STEP 2 Squeeze the thighs against the outer arms using the adductor group of muscles. The most anterior of this group are the adductors longus and brevis, which also synergize hip flexion. The most posterior and the largest of the group is the adductor magnus. The secondary action of this muscle is extension of the hip. Accordingly, when the hip is flexed, some of its fibers are stretching, which places the adductor magnus at a slight biomechanical disadvantage for contributing to adduction of the femurs.

Engage the triceps to straighten the elbows and the anterior and lateral deltoids to flex and abduct the shoulders. These actions are necessary to lift the body and provide a resistance for the inner thighs to squeeze against. Co-contracting these muscles connects the upper and lower appendicular skeletons to form a structural bandha that stabilizes the pose.

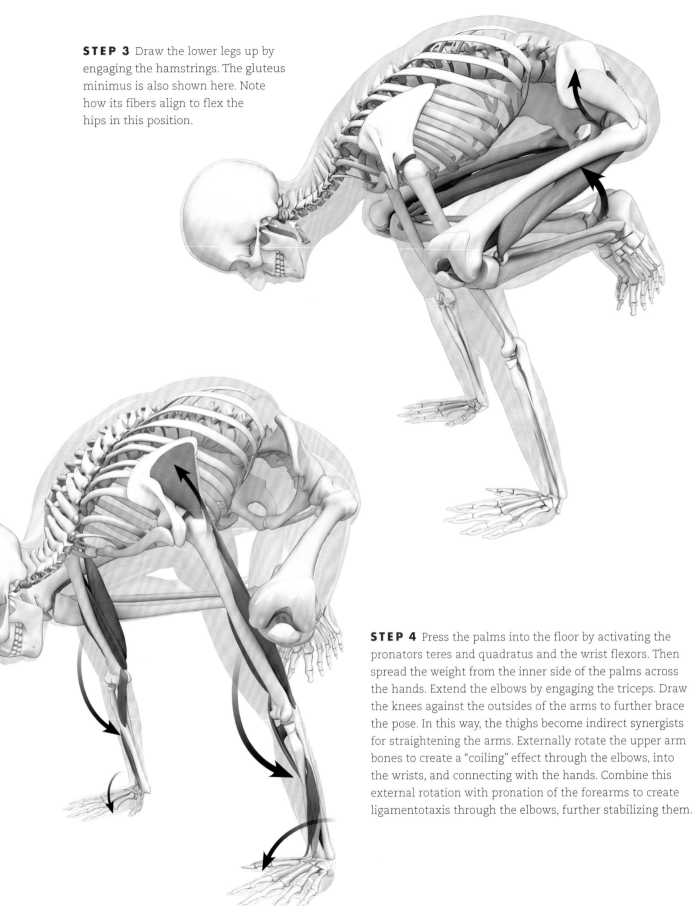

STEP 3 Draw the lower legs up by engaging the hamstrings. The gluteus minimus is also shown here. Note how its fibers align to flex the hips in this position.

STEP 4 Press the palms into the floor by activating the pronators teres and quadratus and the wrist flexors. Then spread the weight from the inner side of the palms across the hands. Extend the elbows by engaging the triceps. Draw the knees against the outsides of the arms to further brace the pose. In this way, the thighs become indirect synergists for straightening the arms. Externally rotate the upper arm bones to create a "coiling" effect through the elbows, into the wrists, and connecting with the hands. Combine this external rotation with pronation of the forearms to create ligamentotaxis through the elbows, further stabilizing them.

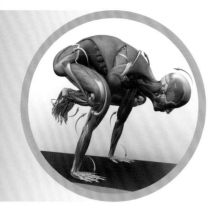

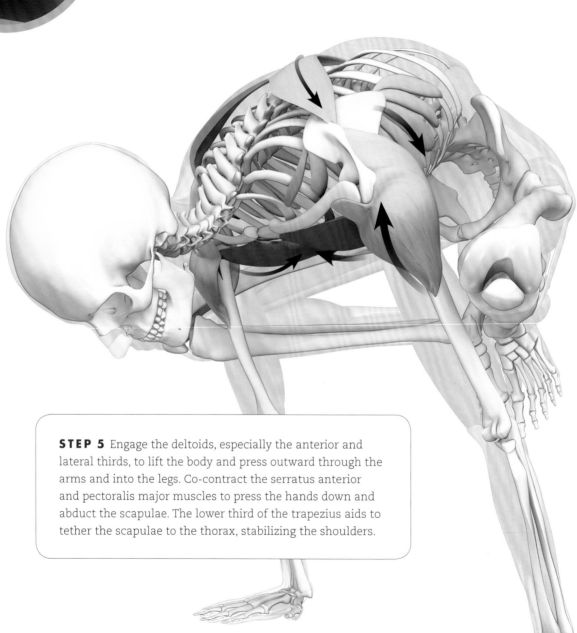

STEP 5 Engage the deltoids, especially the anterior and lateral thirds, to lift the body and press outward through the arms and into the legs. Co-contract the serratus anterior and pectoralis major muscles to press the hands down and abduct the scapulae. The lower third of the trapezius aids to tether the scapulae to the thorax, stabilizing the shoulders.

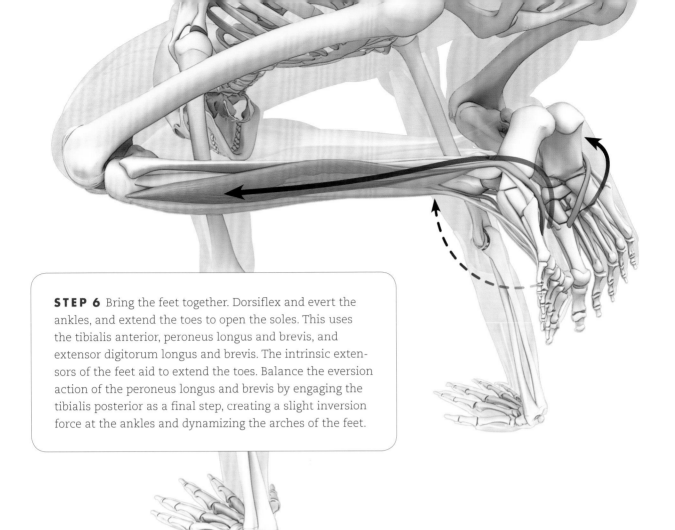

STEP 6 Bring the feet together. Dorsiflex and evert the ankles, and extend the toes to open the soles. This uses the tibialis anterior, peroneus longus and brevis, and extensor digitorum longus and brevis. The intrinsic extensors of the feet aid to extend the toes. Balance the eversion action of the peroneus longus and brevis by engaging the tibialis posterior as a final step, creating a slight inversion force at the ankles and dynamizing the arches of the feet.

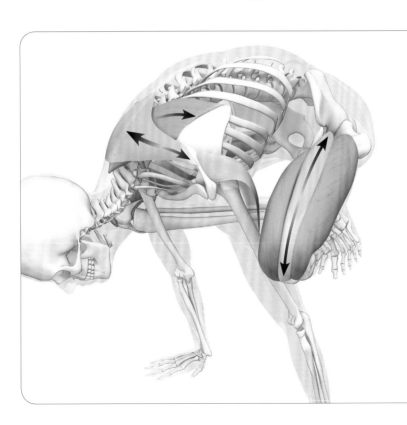

SUMMARY The main stretch in this pose is of the rhomboids and middle third of the trapezius, due to abduction of the scapulae. The serratus and pectoralis muscles create reciprocal inhibition of the rhomboids and trapezius, resulting in some degree of relaxation in the stretch. Flexing the shoulders stretches the posterior deltoids. Flexing the knees stretches the quadriceps. All of the synergists of the pose are strengthened and the shoulders are stabilized. Proprioception and balance improve in this and similar postures.

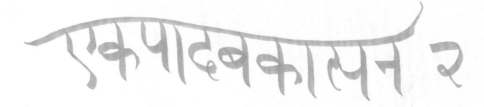

EKA PADA
BAKASANA II
ONE-LEGGED CRANE POSE VERSION II

EKA PADA BAKASANA II IS AN ADVANCED VARIATION OF BAKASANA. NOTICE HOW THE various components of the pose interact with each other. For example, both hips flex and one knee straightens while the other is bent. The position of the straight leg is similar to Kurmasana (Tortoise Pose), and the combination of both legs is like Triang Mukhaikapada Paschimottanasana. Similar to Kurmasana, the straight leg is drawn in against the upper arm, or even the shoulder, creating balance and stability. The straight-leg thigh braces the shoulder while stretching the muscles at the back of the leg and the buttocks. This position strengthens the quadriceps, which then provide feedback through reciprocal inhibition to relax the hamstrings. At the same time, the center of gravity shifts slightly forward and to the straight-leg side, projecting outside the confines of the body.

Imagine an axis of rotation at the center of the chest and balance the body around it. Squeeze the thighs toward the arms, and co-activate the straight-leg quadriceps and bent-leg hamstrings. Engage mula bandha to contract the pubococcygeus muscle and nutate the sacrum. Combine this with engaging the abdominals to tuck the tailbone under. This can be used to counterbalance the forward momentum of the body. Once you attain stability, engage the triceps and chest muscles to lift the torso upwards.

BASIC JOINT POSITIONS

- The hips flex and adduct.
- One knee flexes and the other extends.
- The straight-leg ankle plantar flexes, the foot everts, and the toes extend.
- The bent-leg ankle dorsiflexes, the foot everts, and the toes extend.
- The trunk flexes.

- The shoulders flex, adduct, and externally rotate.
- The elbows extend.
- The forearms pronate.
- The wrists extend.
- The cervical spine extends.

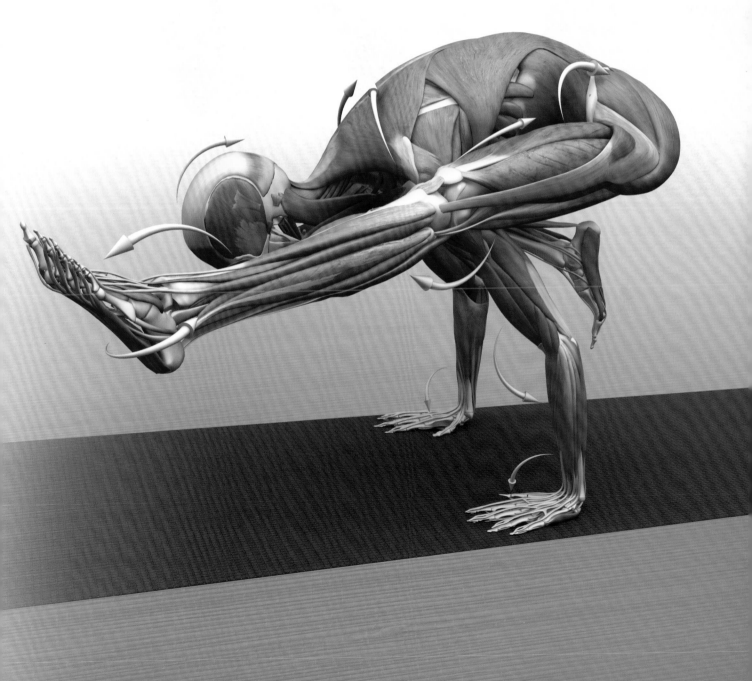

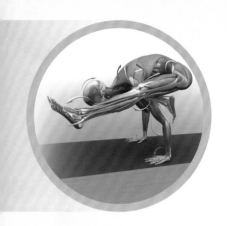

Eka Pada Bakasana II
Preparation

The preparation for this pose is similar to Bakasana; however, you may wish to take the general form of Kurmasana and Triang Mukhaikapada Paschimottanasana before going up into the balance. Eka Pada Bakasana II requires flexibility in the hips and length in the hamstrings. The forward bends, with facilitated stretches of the hamstrings and gluteals, help to prepare for this.

Press the hands into the floor with the knees on either side of the arms. Squeeze in with the legs and out with the arms to feel the muscle groups that activate in the pose. Tilt forward onto the tip-toes, contract the abdominals, and tuck the tailbone. Which way does your weight shift—forward or back? At this point, you might try straightening the leg (before coming up into a balance). When you come out, rest for a moment in Uttanasana before going on. This gives the unconscious brain an opportunity to develop circuitry to more efficiently perform the pose. Then come up onto the toes again and lean forward into Bakasana. Ease one leg toward full extension by flexing the hip and engaging the quadriceps. Squeeze the thighs into the arms. Reverse the process to ease out of the pose by bending the knee back to Bakasana and then tilting the body weight back and down onto the toes. Come up and relax in Uttanasana.

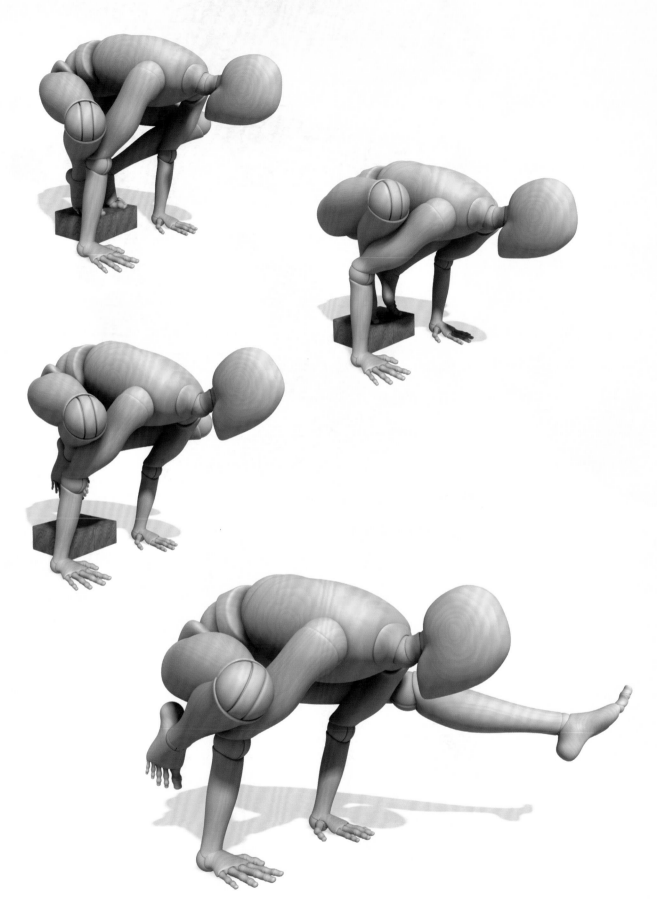

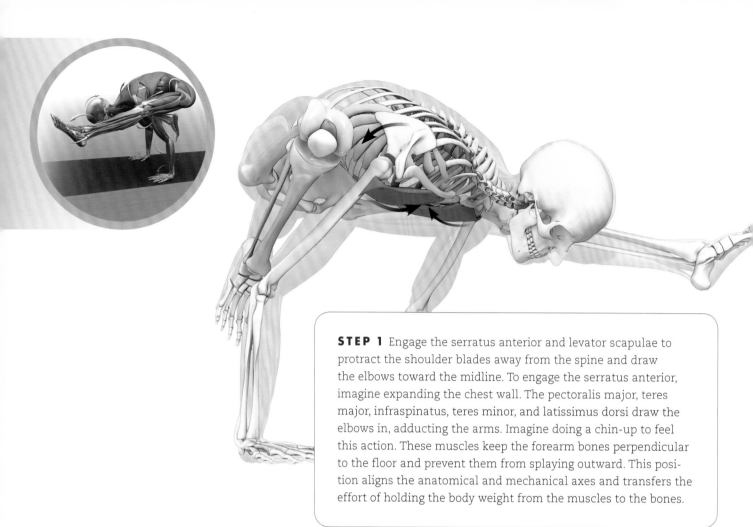

STEP 1 Engage the serratus anterior and levator scapulae to protract the shoulder blades away from the spine and draw the elbows toward the midline. To engage the serratus anterior, imagine expanding the chest wall. The pectoralis major, teres major, infraspinatus, teres minor, and latissimus dorsi draw the elbows in, adducting the arms. Imagine doing a chin-up to feel this action. These muscles keep the forearm bones perpendicular to the floor and prevent them from splaying outward. This position aligns the anatomical and mechanical axes and transfers the effort of holding the body weight from the muscles to the bones.

STEP 2 Press the hands into the mat using the pronators teres and quadratus, as well as the wrist flexors. This balances the external rotation forces that the infraspinatus and teres minor muscles produce to keep the elbows drawing in (as described in Step 1). Engage the triceps to attempt to straighten the elbows. In addition to extending the elbows, the long head of the triceps (which originates from the scapula) stabilizes the shoulder blade; this synergizes the muscles in Step 1. Lift the torso by contracting the deltoid muscles at the fronts of the shoulders. A cue for this is to imagine raising the arms overhead. Note how the muscles and bones interconnect from the hands through the elbows and into the shoulders in a coiling fashion.

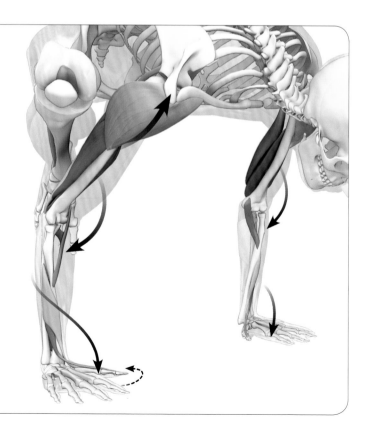

STEP 3 Contract the psoas to flex the hip. Visualize the gluteus minimus engaging to synergize this action. Activate the hamstrings to flex the knee. This tilts the pelvis back and down by pulling on the ischial tuberosities and counters the anterior tilt of the pelvis produced by the contracting psoas. Co-activating antagonist muscles can be used to stabilize a region—in this case, the pelvis. Evert the ankle and dorsiflex the foot by engaging the peronei and extensor digitorum. You can try this before entering the pose to see how it works. These actions create ligamentotaxis (the pull of ligaments on bones) and activate the arches of the feet. Engage the extensors digitorum longus and brevis to extend the toes. Counter eversion of the ankle by contracting the tibialis posterior muscle. This dynamizes the arch of the foot and stabilizes the bones of the lower leg.

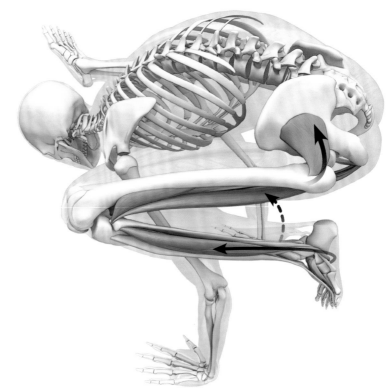

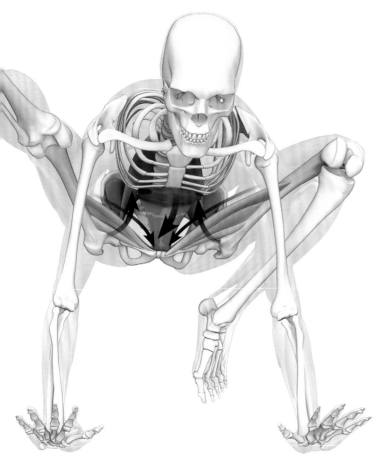

STEP 4 Draw the pelvis upward by engaging the abdominals, especially the rectus abdominis. Combine this with actively flexing the hips from the tops of the thighs by contracting the psoas and its synergists—the pectineus and adductors longus and brevis. The synergists of the psoas combine to squeeze the legs into the upper arms. Look at the matrix of interactions between the various muscle groups and the coupled movements of the hips, pelvis, and spine in this pose.

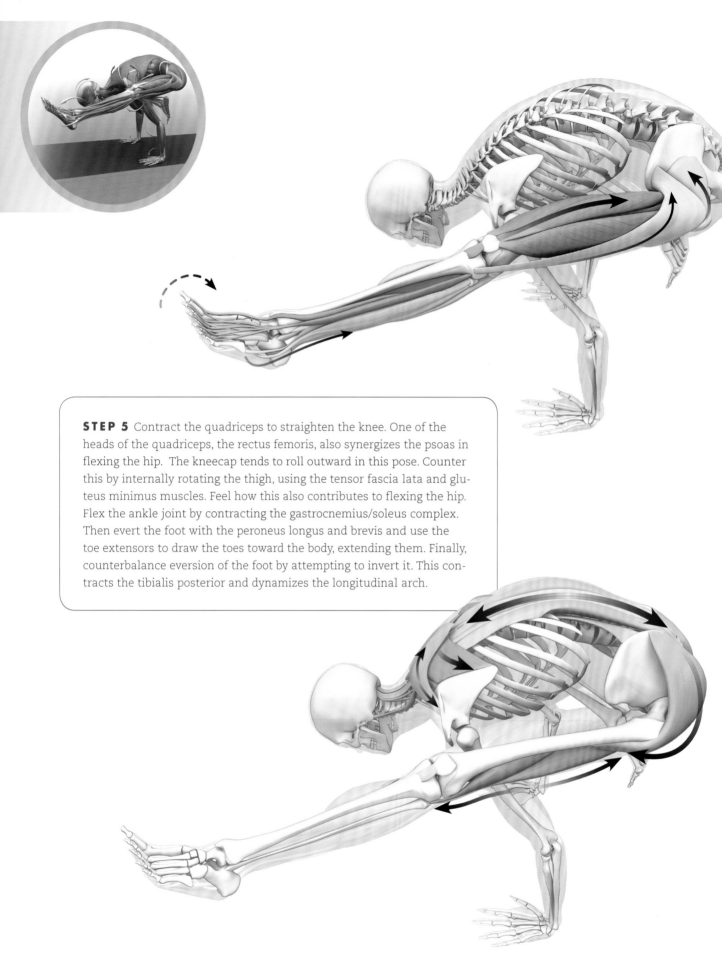

STEP 5 Contract the quadriceps to straighten the knee. One of the heads of the quadriceps, the rectus femoris, also synergizes the psoas in flexing the hip. The kneecap tends to roll outward in this pose. Counter this by internally rotating the thigh, using the tensor fascia lata and gluteus minimus muscles. Feel how this also contributes to flexing the hip. Flex the ankle joint by contracting the gastrocnemius/soleus complex. Then evert the foot with the peroneus longus and brevis and use the toe extensors to draw the toes toward the body, extending them. Finally, counterbalance eversion of the foot by attempting to invert it. This contracts the tibialis posterior and dynamizes the longitudinal arch.

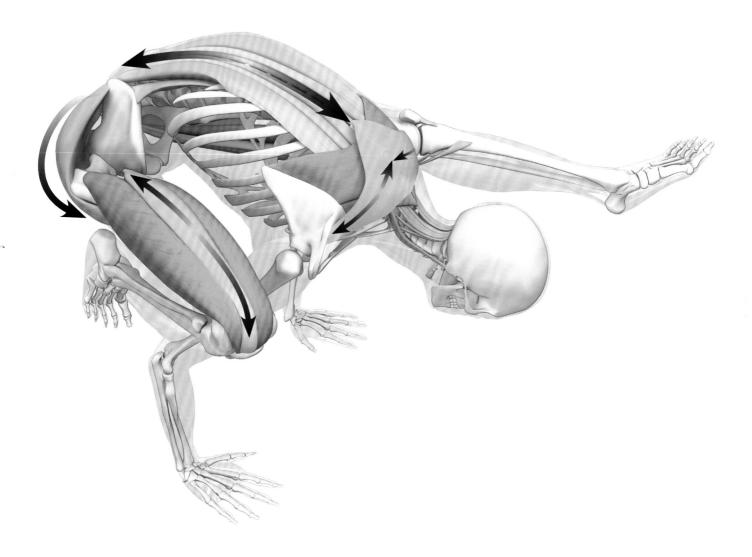

SUMMARY Straightening the knee lengthens the hamstrings. Contracting the quadriceps produces reciprocal inhibition of these same muscles. This helps the hamstrings relax into the stretch. Flexing the hip stretches the gluteus maximus and adductor magnus (on the posterior inner thigh). Flexing the trunk lengthens the erector spinae and quadratus lumborum muscles. Protracting (abducting) the scapulae lengthens the rhomboids and middle third of the trapezius. Flexing the knee stretches the quadriceps. All of this blends balance training with strengthening of the shoulder girdle muscles while creating length in the posterior kinetic chain.

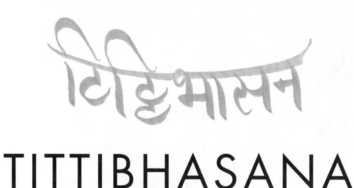

TITTIBHASANA

FIREFLY POSE

IN TITTIBHASANA, BOTH HIPS FLEX AND THE KNEES EXTEND. THE INNER LEGS PRESS against the arms, connecting the upper and lower extremities and bracing the elbows. Joining the inner thighs and upper arms draws strength from the core of the pelvic and shoulder girdles for balancing in the pose. Tittibhasana is a symmetrical posture that shifts the center of gravity forward from Bakasana. The forward extension through the feet is constrained backward by the outward push of the arms against the thighs. There is also an upward lift of the torso against the downward pull of gravity. Fine adjustments can be made by flexing and extending the ankles. For example, pointing the feet projects the center of gravity forward. Feel how this affects the distribution of weight in the hands. Simultaneously flex the hips and trunk. This action tilts the legs upward. Link this with squeezing the thighs into the arms.

This is an advanced pose. You should be adept in practicing Kurmasana before attempting it, as it requires significant flexibility in the back and hamstrings. See the Facilitated Stretch section on Kurmasana for tips (page 15). Additionally, you should be comfortable performing Bakasana and Chaturanga Dandasana to ensure adequate arm strength and balance for Tittibhasana.

BASIC JOINT POSITIONS

- The hips flex and adduct.
- The knees extend.
- The ankles plantar flex.
- The feet evert.
- The toes flex.
- The trunk flexes.

- The shoulders flex, adduct, and externally rotate.
- The forearms pronate.
- The wrists extend.
- The cervical spine extends.

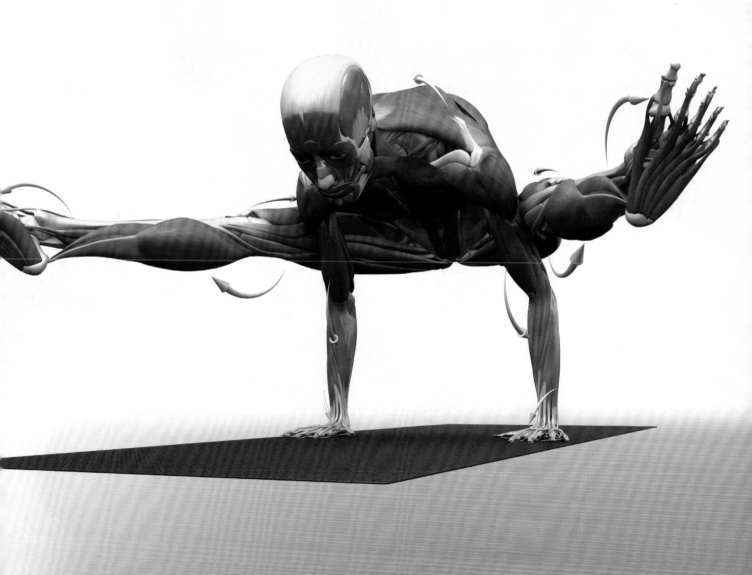

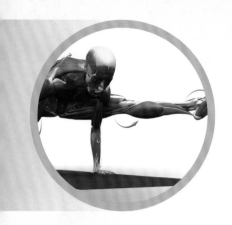

Tittibhasana Preparation

Use the preparation for Bakasana. Squeeze the knees tightly into the sides of the arms. Once you achieve balance in this pose, focus on contracting the quadriceps to slowly extend one knee; keep the other leg pressed in against the arm. Then focus on the quadriceps of the other leg to slowly extend that knee. You can also extend both knees at the same time from Bakasana.

Alternatively, you can raise the body from Kurmasana into Tittibhasana. In either preparation, remember to squeeze the thighs into the arms by flexing and adducting the hips. The higher up on the arms you can get the better.

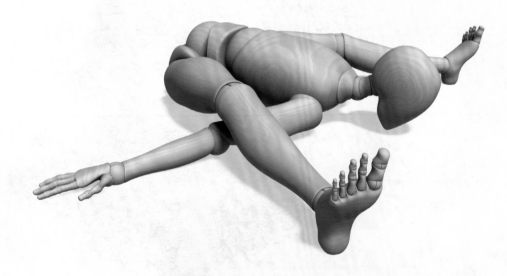

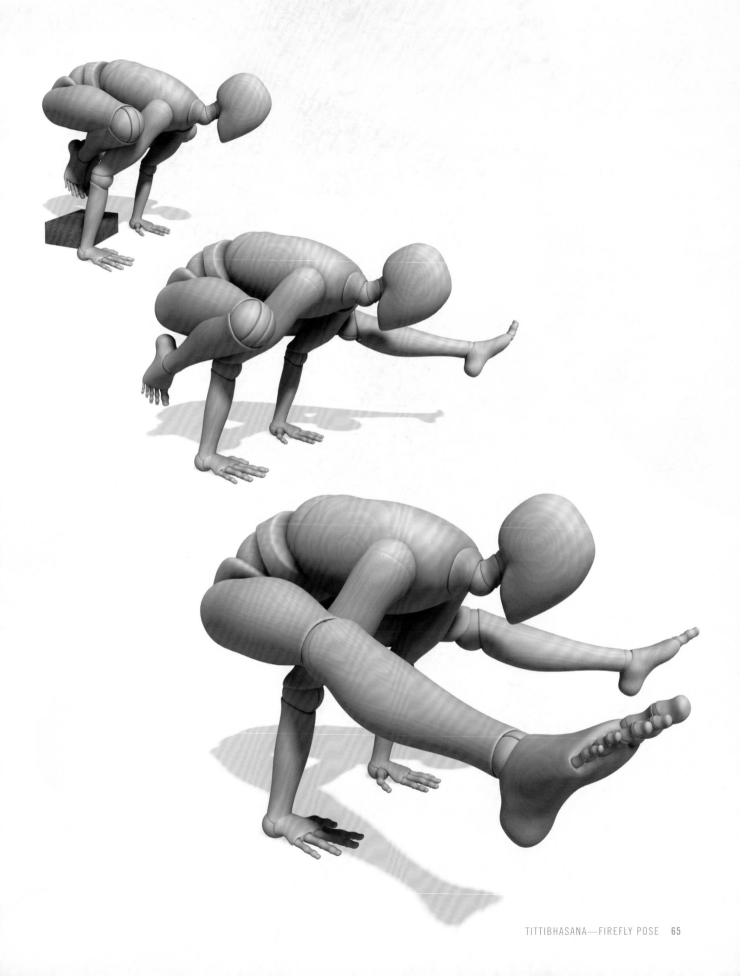

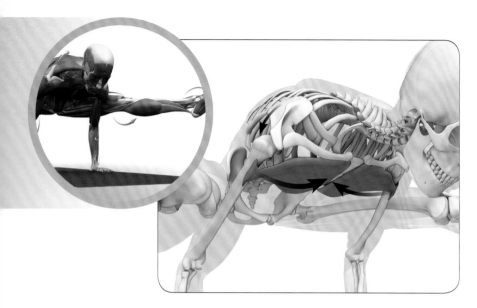

STEP 1 Adduct the humeri and draw the forearms perpendicular to the floor; protract (abduct) the shoulder blades. These actions are the result of firmly engaging the pectoralis major, teres major, latissimus dorsi, long head of the triceps (see Step 2), and coracobrachialis muscles. If you press your hand into a wall and try to draw the hand across your body, you can feel these muscles activating with the other hand. Together with the pectoralis major and minor, the serratus anterior protracts the shoulder blades and draws them away from the midline.

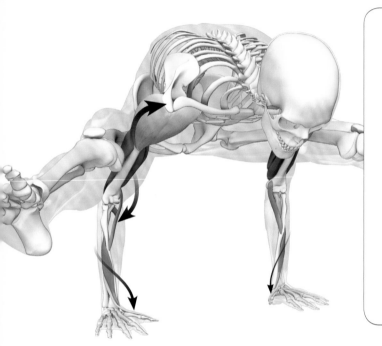

STEP 2 Engage the pronators teres and quadratus to press the hands into the mat. Spread the weight evenly across the palms using the flexors carpi radialis and ulnaris to flex the wrists. Work your way up the arms by engaging the triceps to extend the elbows and stabilize the shoulders. Press the body upwards by activating the anterior and lateral deltoids. Finally, externally rotate the shoulders. Remember that the deltoids are divided into three sections. Use the anterior section to lift the torso up and the lateral section to press the arms outward against the knees. Contract the infraspinatus and teres minor muscles to externally rotate the upper arms; this stabilizes the elbows and prevents them from splaying outward. Eccentrically contract the posterior third of the deltoids to assist in this action.

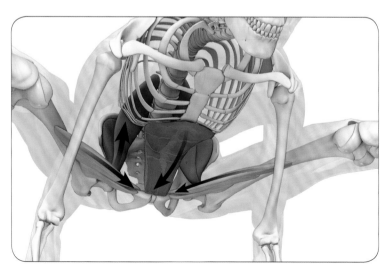

STEP 3 Engage the psoas to flex the hips at the pelvis and lift the legs into the air from the pelvic core. Contract the pectineus and adductors longus and brevis to synergize this action and squeeze the legs into the arms. Activate the abdominals to draw the pubic symphysis upwards; this feels like drawing inward from the lower abdomen, below the navel. Engaging the abdominals reciprocally inhibits the erector spinae and other back muscles, allowing them to lengthen into the stretch.

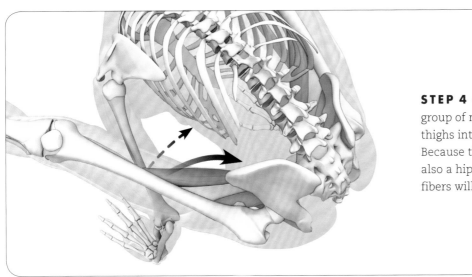

STEP 4 Contract the adductor group of muscles to press the thighs into the upper arms. Because the adductor magnus is also a hip extensor, many of its fibers will stretch in Tittibhasana.

STEP 5 Straighten the knees by engaging the quadriceps. This creates reciprocal inhibition of the hamstrings, allowing them to relax into the stretch. The rectus femoris crosses the hip joint (it is polyarticular) and thus synergizes the psoas muscle in flexing the hips. The gluteus minimus and tensor fascia lata muscles also flex and internally rotate the femurs in this position, counteracting the tendency of the stretching gluteus maximus to externally rotate the thighs.

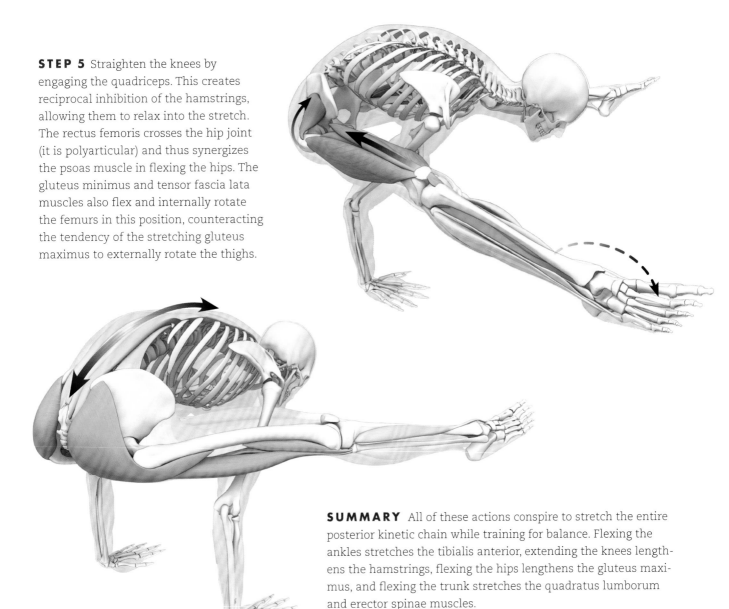

SUMMARY All of these actions conspire to stretch the entire posterior kinetic chain while training for balance. Flexing the ankles stretches the tibialis anterior, extending the knees lengthens the hamstrings, flexing the hips lengthens the gluteus maximus, and flexing the trunk stretches the quadratus lumborum and erector spinae muscles.

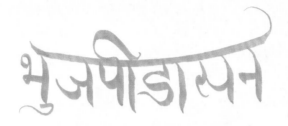

BHUJAPIDASANA

SHOULDER-PRESSING POSE

BHUJAPIDASANA HAS MANY SIMILAR JOINT ACTIONS TO THOSE FOUND IN Tittibhasana, except here the ankles are crossed and the knees are flexed. As with Tittibhasana, Kurmasana can be used to prepare the hips and back for the pose. Ideally, the legs are as high up as possible on the arms, with the weight of the body balanced over the hands. A great deal of flexibility must be attained in the lower back and gluteals to perform this posture. There should also be sufficient external rotation of the hips (meaning length of the internal rotators).

Press up into the pose by straightening the elbows while squeezing the legs around the arms. The thighs form a bandha, or a "lock," where they join with the arms. The contact point where the ankles cross forms another bandha. Attempting to pull the feet apart augments this lock, strengthening the abductors of the hips. Alternatively, you can bend the knees and use the thighs and calves to squeeze the arms (while at the same time attempting to straighten the elbows).

BASIC JOINT POSITIONS

- The hips flex and adduct.
- The knees flex.
- The ankles dorsiflex.
- The feet evert.
- The toes extend.

- The trunk flexes.
- The shoulders flex, adduct, and externally rotate.
- The wrists extend.
- The cervical spine extends.

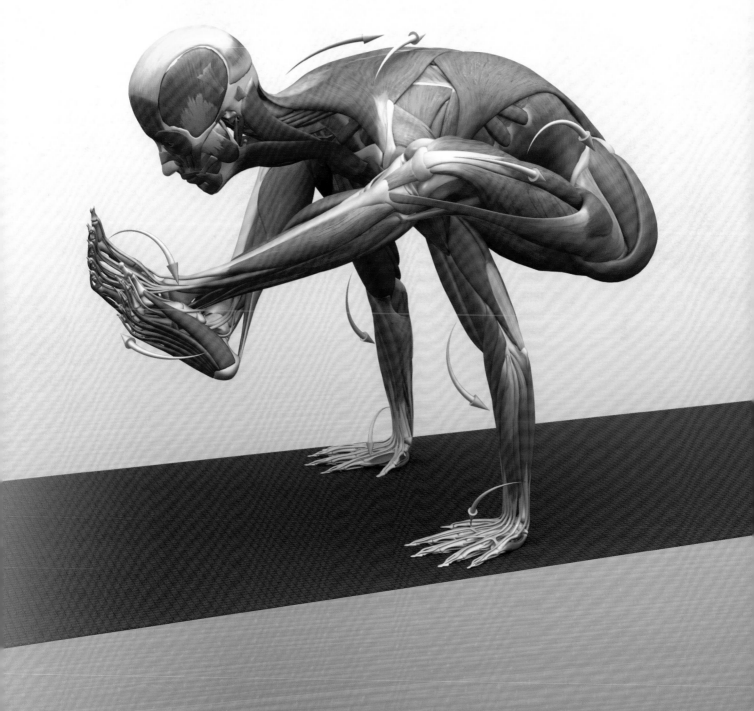

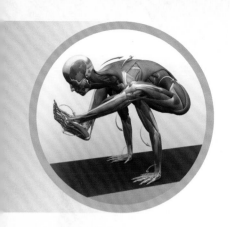

Bhujapidasana Preparation

Gain flexibility in the hips by stretching the internal rotators with cradle stretch, as shown. Use a facilitated stretch to make this more efficient (protecting the knees at all times). Lengthen and prepare the lower back muscles with poses like Prasarita Padottanasana, Kurmasana, and Uttanasana. Strengthen the wrists and arms with Chaturanga Dandasana and Full Arm Balance.

Begin in Tadasana. Bend forward and place the hands in-between and behind the lower legs. Walk the feet in front of the hands. Then hook them around each other, preferably at the ankles, and lift up. Squeeze the thighs into the arms and straighten the knees, pulling on the lock at the ankles. Then bend the knees and squeeze the arms between the legs. In both variations, contract the triceps to straighten the arms and press them outward into the thighs. Come out by unlocking the feet and placing them back on the floor; stand in Uttanasana. Have a bolster or blanket in front of you in the event that you fall forward in the pose.

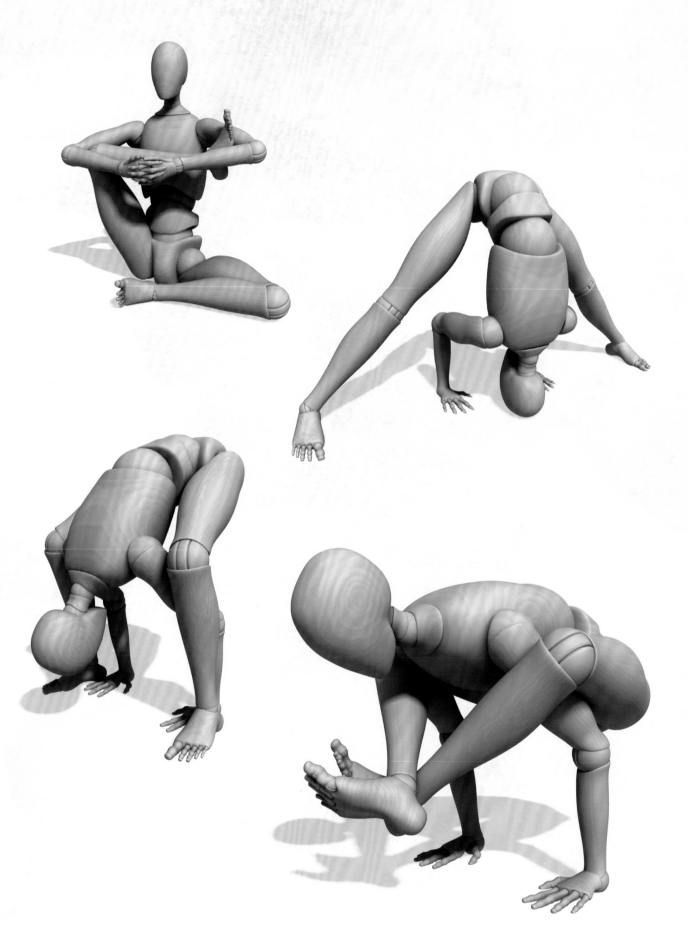

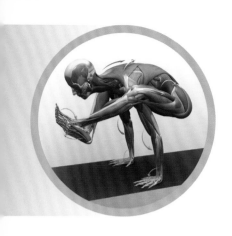

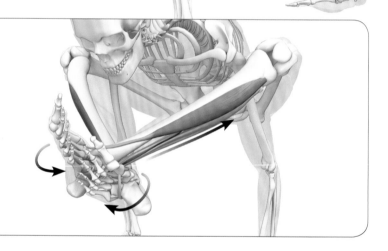

STEP 1 Flex the trunk and hips by contracting the psoas and its synergists (the pectineus, adductors longus and brevis, and sartorius). Engage the rectus abdominis by gently squeezing the stomach muscles to further stabilize the pose.

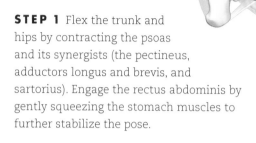

STEP 2 Hook one foot over the other. Then lock the feet by activating the tibialis anterior muscles (draw the tops of the feet toward the shins). Evert the ankles by tilting the outer edges of the feet upward. The peroneus longus and brevis create this action. Then combine the lock at the ankles with the variations described in Steps 4 and 5.

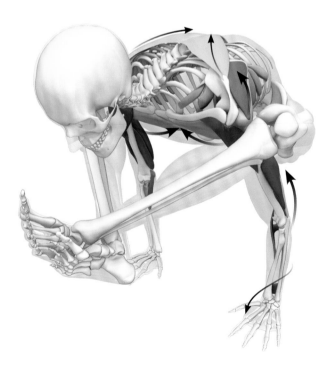

STEP 3 Press the mounds at the base of the index fingers into the mat by pronating the forearms with the pronators teres and quadratus. Lift the body up by engaging the triceps to straighten the elbows. Straightening the elbows produces an outward resistance against the thighs, creating one-half of the lock, with the other half created by the legs. Then use the anterior and lateral deltoids to forward flex the shoulders (as if you were lifting the hands overhead).

Contract the pectoralis major at the front of the chest to add to and stabilize the lift. The serratus anterior will automatically activate and abduct the scapulae away from the midline of the back, tethering the shoulder blades in place. A cue for this is to imagine pressing the hands against a wall while visualizing this muscle engaging.

Finally, externally rotate the shoulders by contracting the infraspinatus and teres minor muscles, as well as the posterior deltoids. This action combines with pronation of the forearms to create a coiling effect down the arms and through the elbows, tightening the ligaments around the elbow joints (ligamentotaxis). This further stabilizes the arms in the pose.

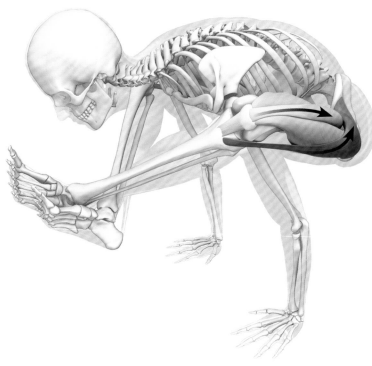

STEP 4 Attempt to straighten the knees by contracting the quadriceps. This is one variation that can be used to create a bandha where the arms and legs meet. The tensor fascia lata contributes to this action in addition to synergizing the psoas in flexing the hips. It also internally rotates the hips, counteracting the pull of the stretching gluteus maximus. Visualize the gluteus minimus contracting to aid the tensor fascia lata.

▶ **STEP 5** Try another variation of Bhujapidasana, where you flex the knees by engaging the hamstrings. This squeezes the arms between the calves and thighs. At the same time, straighten the elbows and note how the arms and legs form a lock, or bandha.

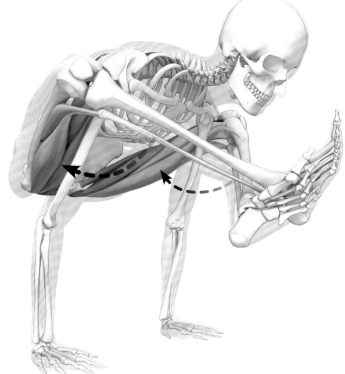

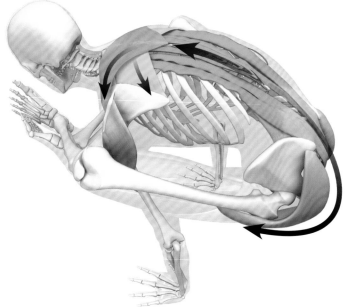

SUMMARY By flexing the trunk and hips, Bhujapidasana stretches the erector spinae and quadratus lumborum muscles of the back, as well as the gluteus maximus. The rhomboids and middle portion of the trapezius also lengthen due to abducting the shoulder blades. Forward flexing the shoulders stretches the posterior deltoids. These muscles also eccentrically contract to externally rotate the shoulders.

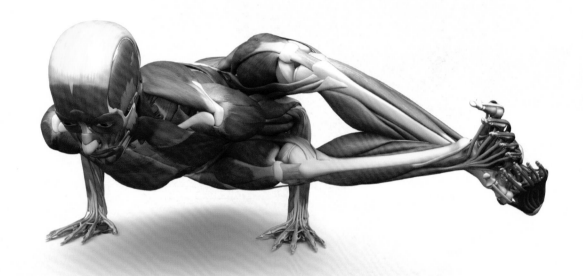

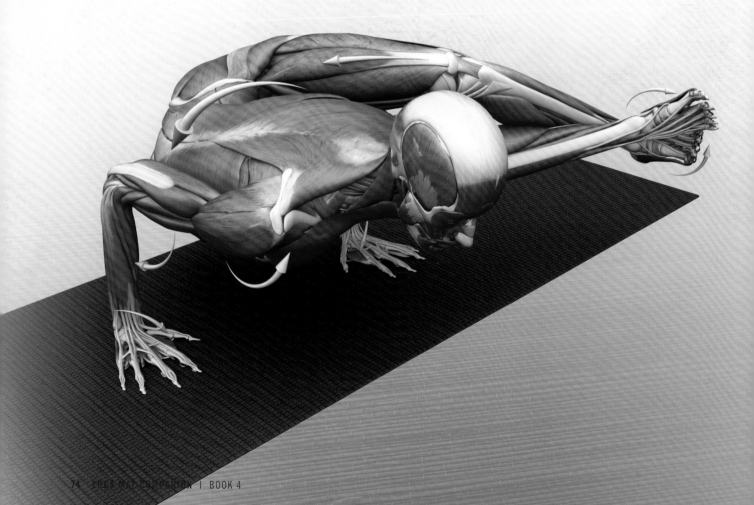

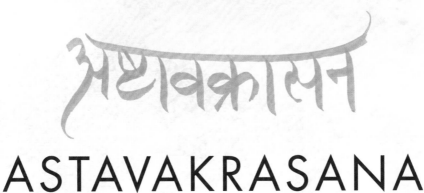

ASTAVAKRASANA

EIGHT-ANGLE POSE

ASTAVAKRASANA COMBINES THE COMPONENTS OF A TWIST AND AN ARM BALANCE. As in Bhujapidasana, the place where the legs wrap around the arm creates the location for a bandha. Look for ways to accentuate the twist in this pose. For example, note how the leg that is on top of the arm hooks its foot under the opposite ankle. Pull up with the top leg to draw the pelvis and lower body deeper into the turn. Then on the other side, press down with the hand and straighten the elbow of the free arm (the arm that doesn't have the legs wrapped around it). This rotates the shoulders and upper body away from the pelvis and deeper into the twist. Look at the muscles that produce these movements and specifically engage them. For example, contract the hip abductors on the upper leg to pull the lower body deeper into the twist. Activate the triceps of the arm that you are attempting to straighten to turn the shoulders and chest. Learn to isolate these muscles and see how engaging them improves the pose. Conversely, observe how this and other yoga poses can be used to increase your awareness of specific muscle groups.

In addition to the twist, a lock is formed where the legs wrap around the arm. Squeeze the arm with the thighs while trying to straighten the elbow. Then attempt to extend the knees. See how the lower leg presses into the forearm, producing a counterforce to the triceps straightening the elbow. These opposing actions create a bandha and stabilize the pose. This takes the effort of the pose into the bones and ligaments, rather than the muscles.

BASIC JOINT POSITIONS

- The hips flex and adduct.
- The knees partly extend.
- The ankles dorsiflex.
- The feet evert.
- The toes extend.
- The trunk flexes and rotates.

- The shoulders adduct and externally rotate.
- The elbows flex.
- The forearms pronate.
- The wrists extend.

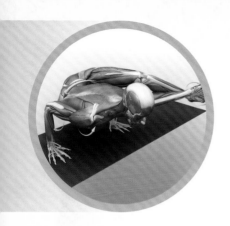

Astavakrasana Preparation

Prepare the torso with Marichyasana III. This not only stretches the trunk, but also lengthens the abductor muscles at the sides of the hips (the tensor fascia lata and gluteus medius). Use poses like the bent-knee version of Supta Padangusthasana to stretch the gluteus maximus and hamstrings. This allows you to get the leg higher up on the shoulder in the final pose. You can also use Kurmasana.

In Astavakrasana, the arms are in a similar position to Chaturanga Dandasana, so practice this pose to strengthen the arms and wrists. Place the elbows in this position and wrap one leg over the shoulder. Cross the feet. Then lean forward into the arms. Practice this a few times to get accustomed to it before coming up into the balance. Then straighten the knees by contracting the quadriceps, squeezing the arm between the thighs. Lean the chest forward and press up into the pose by engaging the triceps, chest muscles, and abdominals. Eventually try the variation in which you straighten both the arms and the legs. Bring the buttocks back to the floor and release the legs. Rest here for a few breaths. Use a bolster or blanket in front of you to cushion against falling forward.

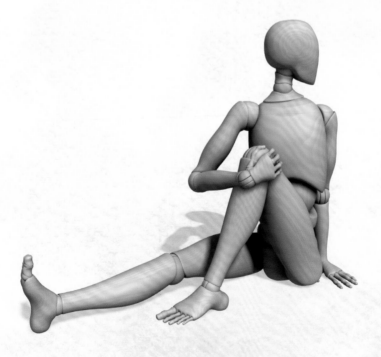

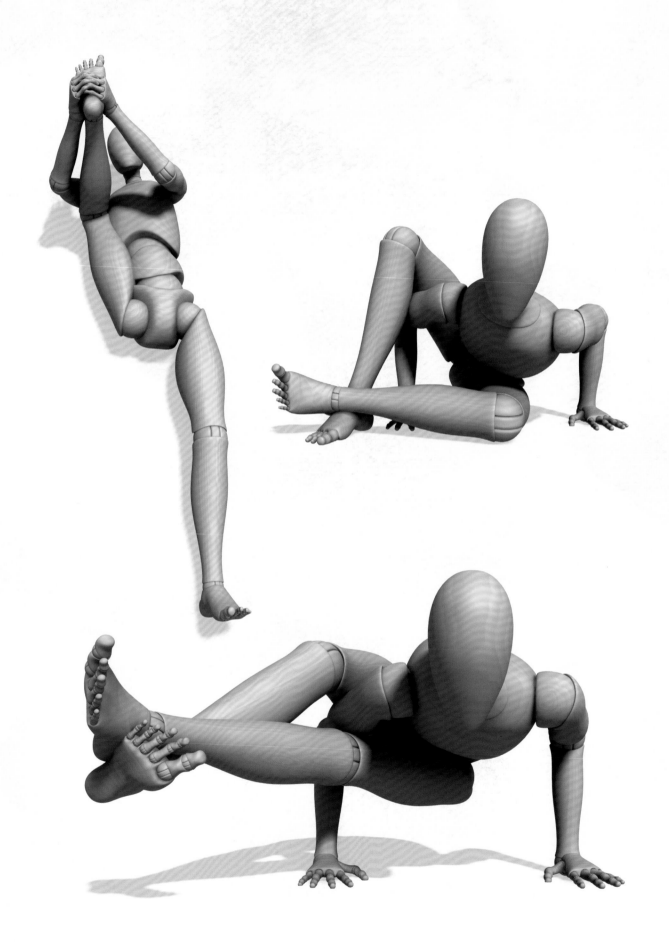

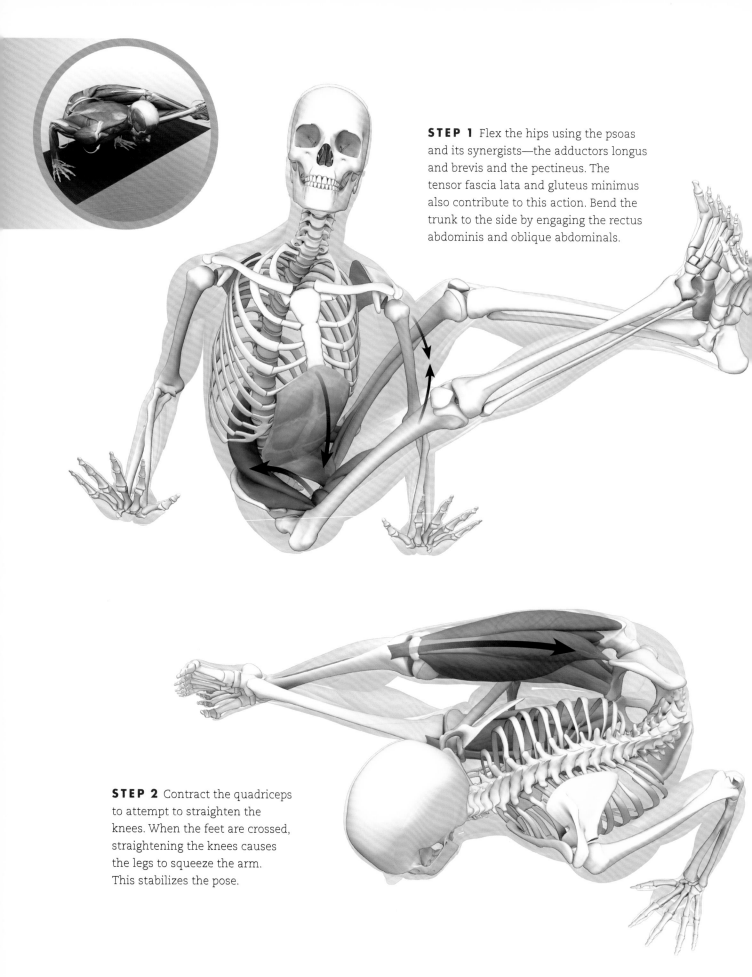

STEP 1 Flex the hips using the psoas and its synergists—the adductors longus and brevis and the pectineus. The tensor fascia lata and gluteus minimus also contribute to this action. Bend the trunk to the side by engaging the rectus abdominis and oblique abdominals.

STEP 2 Contract the quadriceps to attempt to straighten the knees. When the feet are crossed, straightening the knees causes the legs to squeeze the arm. This stabilizes the pose.

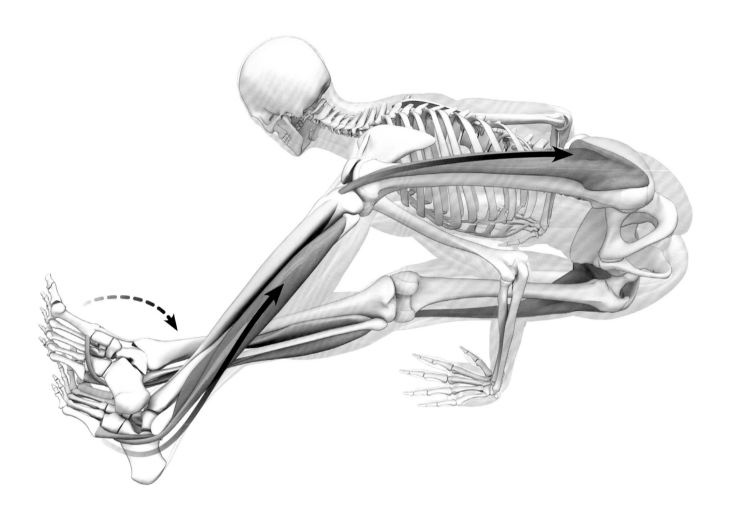

STEP 3 Cross the ankles and evert them by engaging the peroneus longus and brevis muscles at the sides of the lower legs. This locks the ankles together. Then as you straighten the knees, attempt to pull the feet apart. Pull harder on the upper-side leg to engage the gluteus medius and tensor fascia lata more forcefully on this side. This draws the legs deeper into the twist, turning the pelvis in the opposite direction of the shoulders.

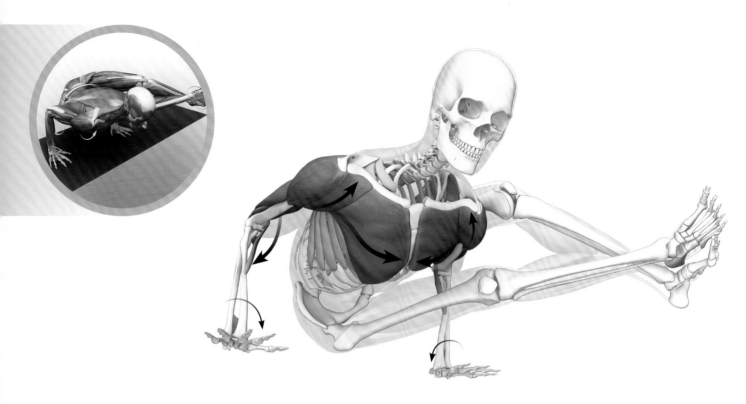

STEP 4 Press the mounds at the base of the index fingers into the mat by contracting the pronators teres and quadratus. Stabilize the elbows by engaging the triceps. Use the pectoralis major to press the body upward, holding the elbows close to the torso. The anterior deltoids aid to lift the trunk. Visualize the serratus anterior pulling the scapulae forward and tethering them to the thorax. These are the same muscles that engage in Chaturanga Dandasana to lift the body from the floor.

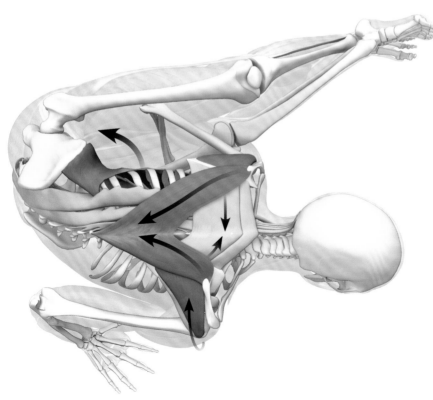

STEP 5 Contract the rhomboids to draw the shoulder blades toward the midline. Engage the infraspinatus, teres minor, and posterior deltoids to externally rotate the shoulders. This works in conjunction with the muscles that pronate the forearms. The cue for engaging these muscles is to press the mounds of the index fingers into the mat. The net effect is a coiling force from the shoulders to the hands that tightens the elbow ligaments (ligamentotaxis).

Engage the upper-side erector spinae and quadratus lumborum to slightly arch the back and laterally flex the trunk. On the upper side, the internal oblique contributes to the lateral flexion. The external oblique rotates the shoulder towards the opposite hip. Feel and visualize these muscles contracting in the pose.

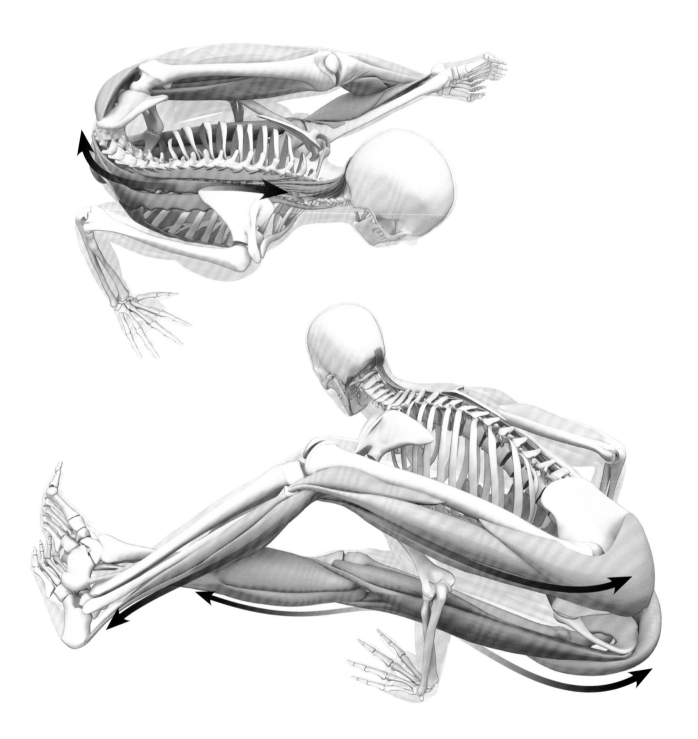

SUMMARY Astavakrasana stretches the lower-side erector spinae and spinal rotators. The gluteus maximus muscles lengthen from flexing the hips. The hamstrings are stretched, as well as the gastrocnemius/soleus complex. Flexing and turning the trunk lengthens the lower-side oblique abdominals and the transversus abdominis.

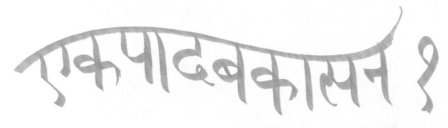

EKA PADA BAKASANA I

ONE-LEGGED CRANE POSE VERSION I

EKA PADA BAKASANA I HAS ONE HIP FLEXING AND THE OTHER EXTENDING. THE KNEE of the rear leg also extends, shifting the center of gravity back. Flex the trunk forward to balance the momentum of the back leg. Note that the main flexor of the forward hip, the psoas, is in a position of active insufficiency. This means that the muscle is already fully contracted, so it cannot generate much additional force to flex the hip. In this situation, the adductor muscles of the bent leg squeeze the inside of the thigh against the upper arm and lever the hip into flexion. The leg tucking up onto the arm combined with the force of the elbow extending creates a focus for balance. Co-contraction of the muscles that hold this position (the muscles of the chest, arm, hip, and leg) is a subplot of the pose that contributes to the whole.

The straight leg is another story. Lifting the leg requires activating the back extensors, gluteals, hamstrings, quadriceps, and calf muscles. The back muscles and ligaments tether the pelvis. The pelvis connects to the gluteal muscles, lifting and rotating the thigh. The quadriceps extend the knee, while the fascia lata, with its contributions from the gluteus maximus and tensor fascia lata, stabilize the knee. The ankle acts as an aileron (or a "wing") to create subtle shifts in the center of gravity by flexing and everting, opening the sole of the foot. Both legs combine to create the main story of the pose—a balance of muscular, ligamentous, and gravitational forces.

BASIC JOINT POSITIONS

- The shoulders flex, adduct, and externally rotate.
- The elbows partly extend.
- The forearms pronate.
- The wrists extend.
- The hip on the bent-knee side flexes and adducts.
- The hip on the extended-knee side extends and internally rotates.
- The bent-leg side ankle dorsiflexes, foot everts, and toes extend.
- The straight-leg side ankle plantar flexes, foot everts, and toes flex.
- The trunk flexes.
- The cervical spine extends.

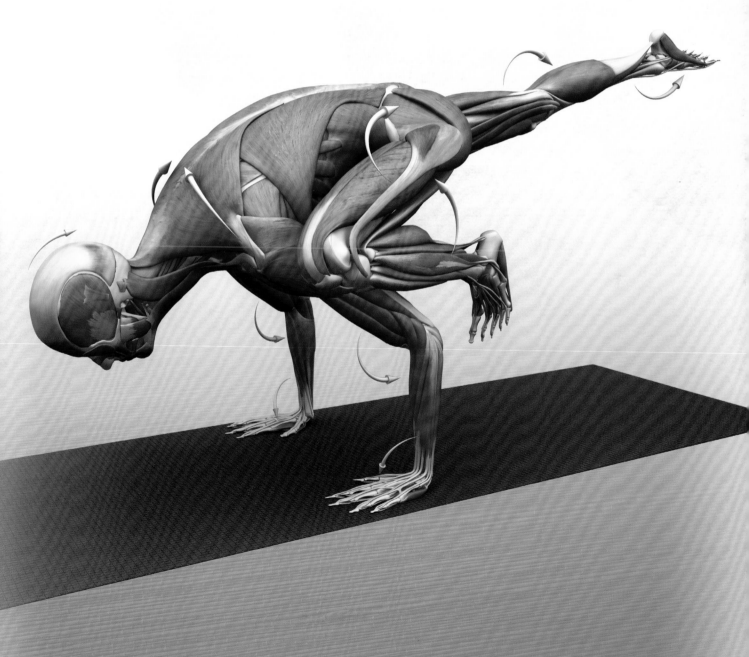

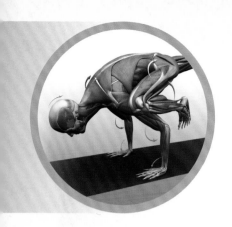

Eka Pada Bakasana I
Preparation

Follow the same preparation as for Bakasana. You can also use the preparatory stretches for Hanumanasana (forward splits) to gain flexibility in the hips for this pose. From the hands and knees position, lift one leg to get a sense for how it feels to extend out through the foot. Focus on the muscles at the back of the leg, the buttocks, and the lower back. Then use a pair of blocks or come directly off the floor to move into Bakasana. Begin to take the pressure off the leg that you will extend, and shift your weight onto the other arm, squeezing that knee and inner thigh tighter against the arm. Lean forward as you straighten the back leg, contracting the buttocks and quadriceps to extend the hip and straighten the knee. Arch the lower back.

Anticipate the change in balance and brace yourself to reverse the process to come out of the pose. Bend the knee and tuck it back onto the upper arm. Create balance between the two sides in Bakasana. Then ease out by tilting backwards and down onto the toes. Flatten the feet and take a relaxed Uttanasana for a moment or two. Then engage the hip and back extensors to stand up.

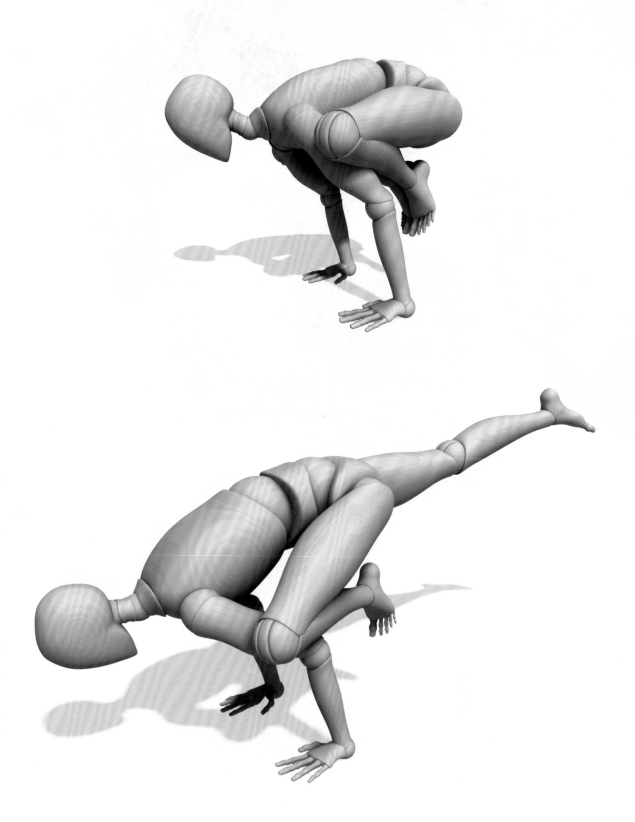

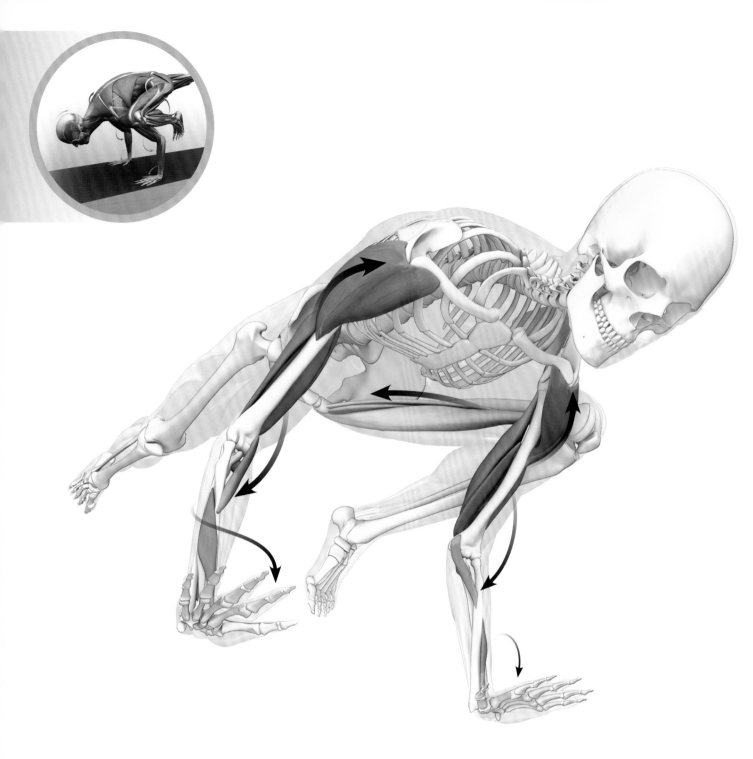

STEP 1 Use the muscles of the arms to create a scaffolding to hold the body up. The torso leans forward to balance the weight of the straight leg, which extends back. Use the wrist flexors to fine tune the forward tilt of the body. Engage the pronators teres and quadratus to pronate the forearms, pressing the mounds at the base of the index fingers into the floor. Then spread the weight evenly across the palms by co-activating the biceps and supinator muscles. Externally rotate the shoulders by contracting the infraspinatus, teres minor, and posterior third of the deltoids. Attempt to straighten the arms. This engages the triceps and stabilizes the elbows. Squeeze the inner thigh of the flexed hip against the arm to brace the elbow, at the same time resisting by pressing the arm against the inner leg. These opposing forces create a bandha. Lift the body up by activating the front and lateral thirds of the deltoids. These are the same muscles that contract when you lift a weight over your head.

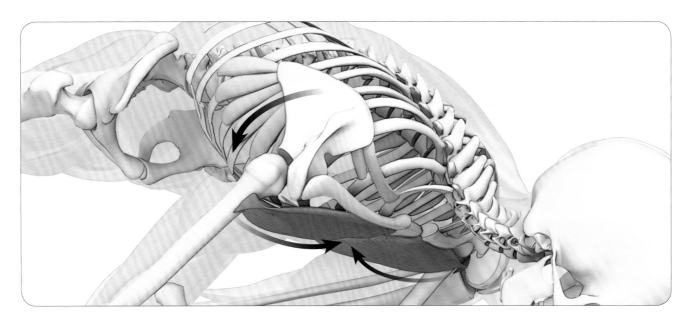

STEP 2 Contract the serratus anterior and pectoralis minor muscles to abduct the shoulder blades away from the spine. Draw the humeri toward the midline to align the upper and lower arms, so that the bones support the body weight as much as possible. The pectoralis major is the prime mover of this action; it also aids the deltoids in lifting the body. The latissimus dorsi and teres major muscles synergize drawing the arms toward the midline. The coracobrachialis of the upper arm synergizes this action. The teres minor and infraspinatus of the rotator cuff externally rotate the humeri. All these actions work together to stabilize the shoulders and arms—the foundation of Eka Pada Bakasana I.

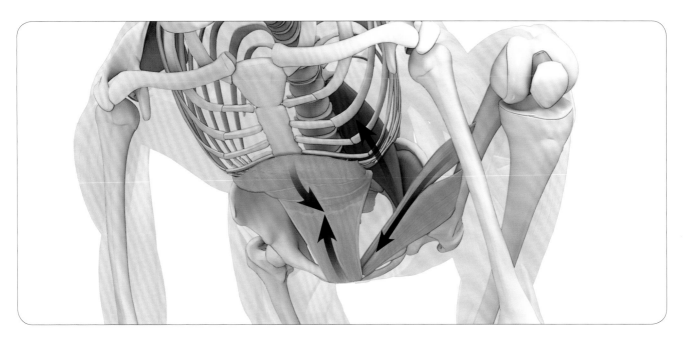

STEP 3 Contract the rectus abdominis to lift the abdominal contents up toward the spine. This muscle attaches to the pubic symphysis. Activating it draws the pubic symphysis upwards, tilting the pelvis into retroversion. This synergizes the action of the straight-leg gluteus maximus and hamstrings, which also retrovert the pelvis. Engage the psoas and quadratus lumborum to flex the hip and slightly arch the lower back. This tilts the pelvis forward, countering the actions of the gluteus maximus and hamstrings. These opposing forces stabilize the core. Contract the adductor group of muscles and the pectineus to indirectly flex the hip by drawing the inner thigh tight against the upper arm.

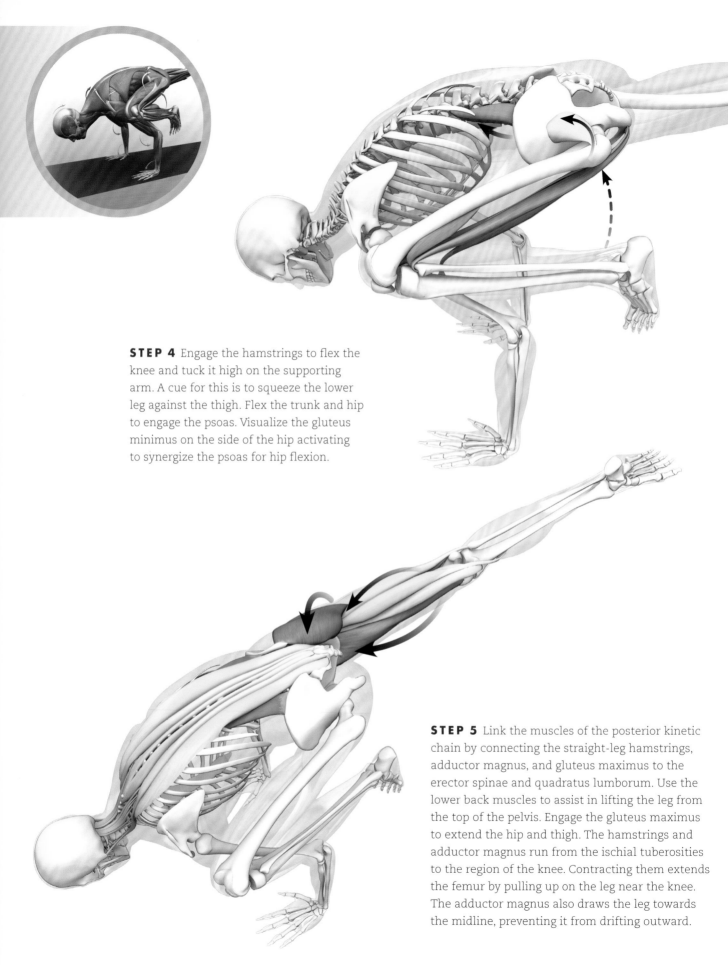

STEP 4 Engage the hamstrings to flex the knee and tuck it high on the supporting arm. A cue for this is to squeeze the lower leg against the thigh. Flex the trunk and hip to engage the psoas. Visualize the gluteus minimus on the side of the hip activating to synergize the psoas for hip flexion.

STEP 5 Link the muscles of the posterior kinetic chain by connecting the straight-leg hamstrings, adductor magnus, and gluteus maximus to the erector spinae and quadratus lumborum. Use the lower back muscles to assist in lifting the leg from the top of the pelvis. Engage the gluteus maximus to extend the hip and thigh. The hamstrings and adductor magnus run from the ischial tuberosities to the region of the knee. Contracting them extends the femur by pulling up on the leg near the knee. The adductor magnus also draws the leg towards the midline, preventing it from drifting outward.

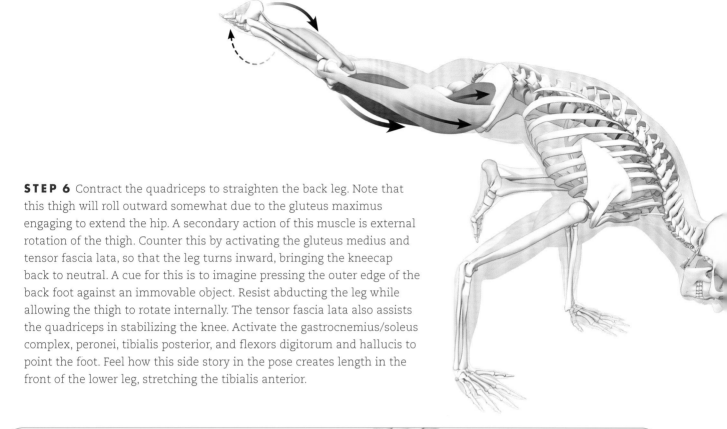

STEP 6 Contract the quadriceps to straighten the back leg. Note that this thigh will roll outward somewhat due to the gluteus maximus engaging to extend the hip. A secondary action of this muscle is external rotation of the thigh. Counter this by activating the gluteus medius and tensor fascia lata, so that the leg turns inward, bringing the kneecap back to neutral. A cue for this is to imagine pressing the outer edge of the back foot against an immovable object. Resist abducting the leg while allowing the thigh to rotate internally. The tensor fascia lata also assists the quadriceps in stabilizing the knee. Activate the gastrocnemius/soleus complex, peronei, tibialis posterior, and flexors digitorum and hallucis to point the foot. Feel how this side story in the pose creates length in the front of the lower leg, stretching the tibialis anterior.

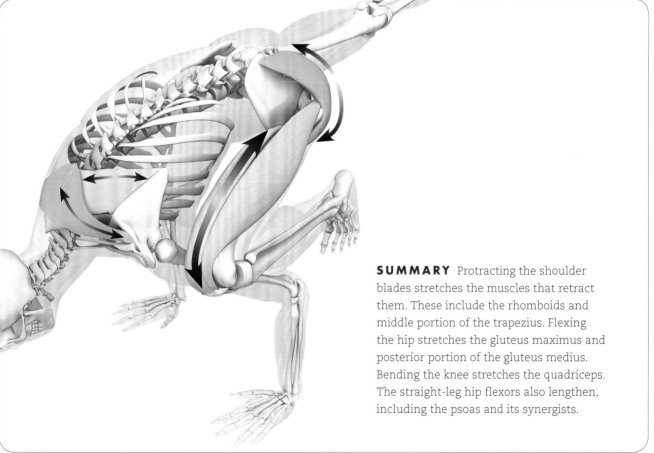

SUMMARY Protracting the shoulder blades stretches the muscles that retract them. These include the rhomboids and middle portion of the trapezius. Flexing the hip stretches the gluteus maximus and posterior portion of the gluteus medius. Bending the knee stretches the quadriceps. The straight-leg hip flexors also lengthen, including the psoas and its synergists.

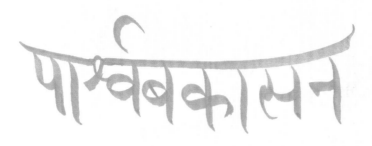

PARSVA BAKASANA

TWISTING CRANE POSE

PARSVA BAKASANA IS A TWISTING VERSION OF BAKASANA, WHEREIN THE CONTACT point between the side of the leg and the arm can be the main focus of the pose. This is the cornerstone for the balance and also a point of leverage for deepening the twist. Several subplots in Parsva Bakasana help to achieve and maintain the final asana. The hips flex to a point of active insufficiency. This means that the prime mover of this action, the psoas, cannot generate much additional force for holding the legs up on the arms because it is already fully contracted. Thus the abdominals combine with the hip flexors to bring the legs onto the arms, and then other muscles are used to lock the legs in place. This creates a fluid synergy between subplots, since the muscles that press the leg into the arm also turn the lower body away from the upper body in the twist. This action then links to the opposite arm, which straightens to turn the chest and upper body. The lumbar spine connects the chest and pelvis. Contracting one side of the abdominals increases the stretch of the other side. Activating the abdominals on the lower side of the body stabilizes the pose by drawing the outer thigh tighter against the arm. This eccentric contraction also stimulates the Golgi tendon organ of the stretching abdominals, causing reflex lengthening of these muscles.

BASIC JOINT POSITIONS

- The shoulders flex, adduct, and externally rotate.
- The elbows extend.
- The forearms pronate.
- The wrists extend.
- The hips flex and adduct.

- The knees flex.
- The ankles dorsiflex.
- The feet evert and the toes extend.
- The trunk flexes and rotates.
- The cervical spine extends.

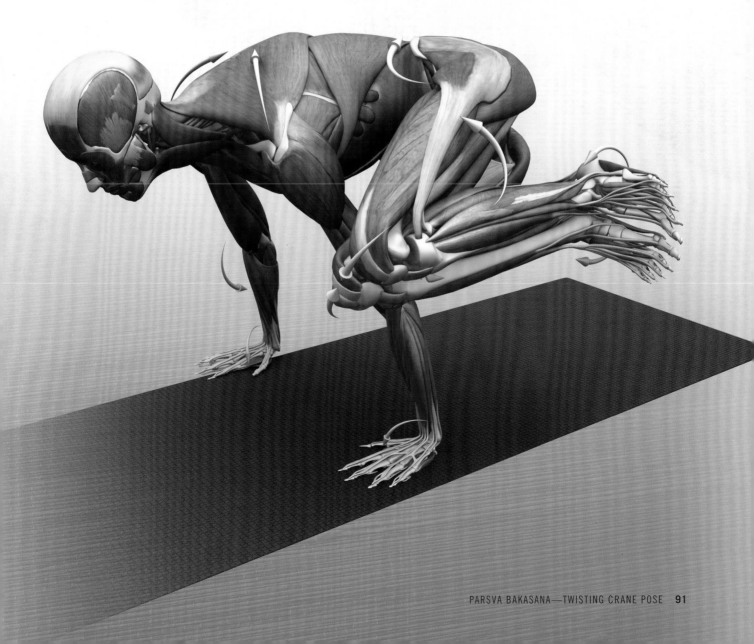

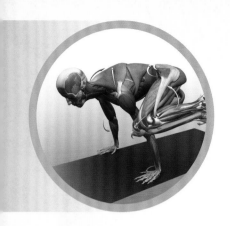

Parsva Bakasana Preparation

Prepare for Parsva Bakasana by practicing the chair twist illustrated here. To further develop the twist, place a block under the heels and squeeze the thighs together at the knees. Then place the hands in prayer position, and press the back of the arm against the side of the thigh to turn the body. Try fixing the thigh and pressing the arm against it; then fix the arm and press the thigh against the arm. Finally, press both the thigh and the arm against each other equally. Feel how each of these actions stretches different parts of the body.

Begin to tilt forward onto the tip-toes. Squeeze the knees together and lift up into the asana. See the muscles section below for how to use biomechanics to create a lock between the knees and keep them pressed together evenly. Connect squeezing the knees together with mula bandha to recruit the muscles of the pelvic floor and cause them to contract more forcefully.

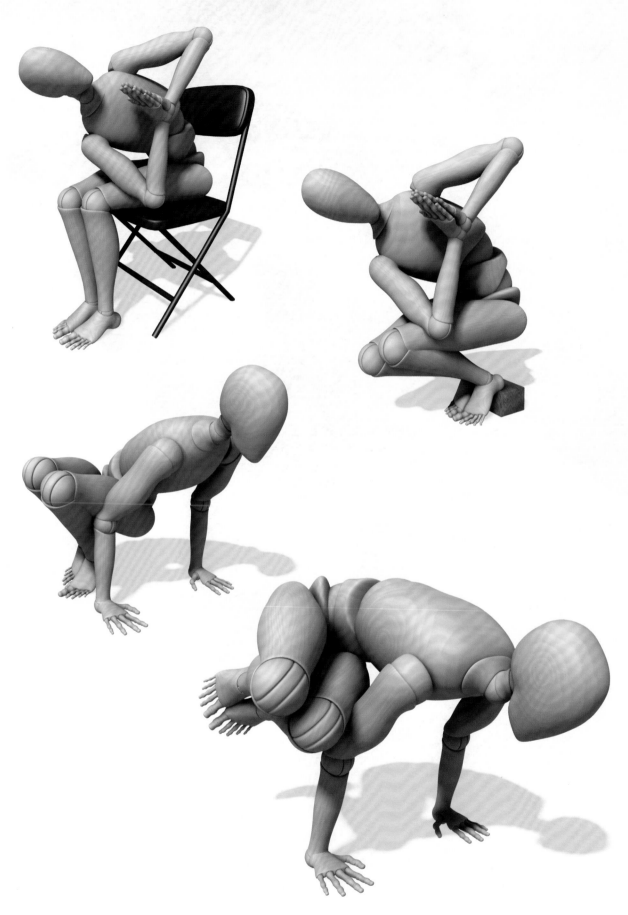

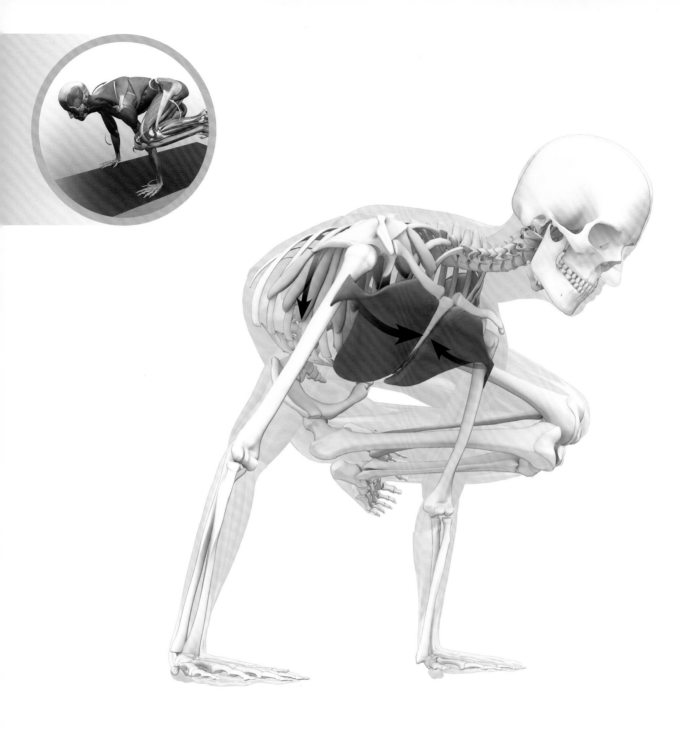

STEP 1 Engage the serratus anterior and pectoralis minor to protract the scapulae away from the midline of the back. Contract the pectoralis major and its synergists to adduct the humeri. All combine to lift the torso and stabilize the shoulders—a key function in the pose. To get a feeling for contracting these muscles, stand facing a wall and press one hand against it, drawing the elbow in toward the side (adducting it). With your other hand, feel the pectoralis major (at the front of the chest) and the teres minor and major (under the arm and on the scapula). Engage these same muscles in the final pose.

STEP 2 Your hands are the foundation. Connect them to the wrists, elbows, and shoulders. Pronate the forearms and press the palms of the hands into the mat, using the pronators teres and quadratus as well as the flexors carpi radialis and ulnaris (wrist flexors). Maintain stability in the hands and wrists and then contract the triceps to lift the body upwards by straightening the elbows. The long head of the triceps originates from the scapula. This means that its contraction contributes to stabilizing the shoulder girdle. Activate the front deltoids to synergize the action of the triceps and pectoralis major in lifting the body. Use the lateral deltoids to press the arm against the thigh, locking the hips into flexion and twisting the torso. Note how the muscles of the arms integrate with those of the shoulder girdle described in Step 1.

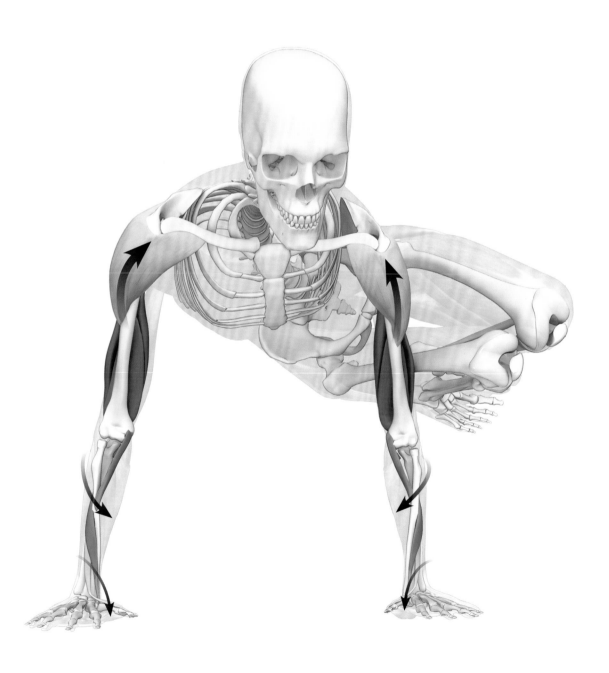

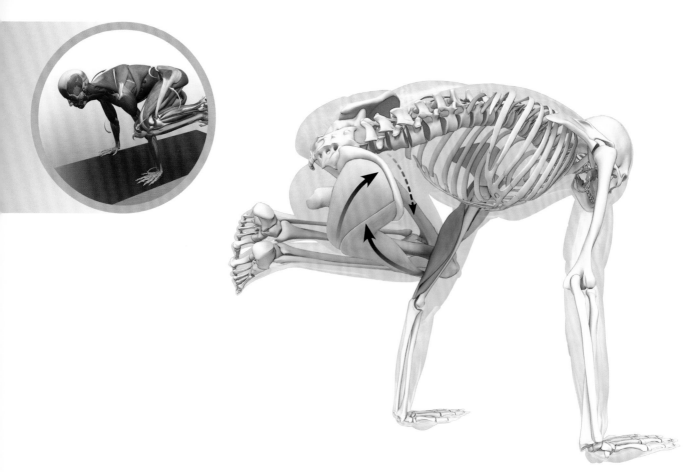

STEP 3 Engage the tensor fascia lata and gluteus medius muscles of the hip to press (abduct) the thigh against the upper arm (above). Squeeze the upper arm against the thigh, using the triceps to straighten the arm and the lateral deltoid to abduct the shoulder outwards (below). These actions create a point of contact that stabilizes the pose and augments the twist.

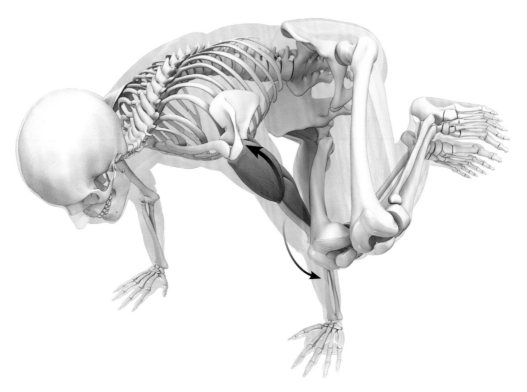

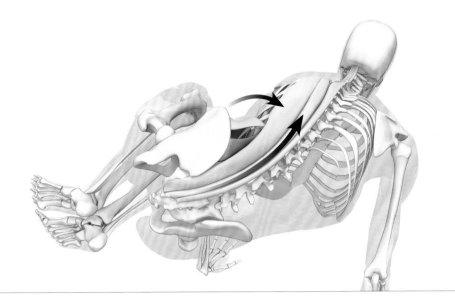

STEP 4 Combine the upper-side back muscles (the erector spinae and spinal rotators) and quadratus lumborum with the oblique abdominals to twist the body. This image illustrates how the spine connects the shoulders and hips in the pose. The oblique abdominals are like sheets of muscle that slide over one another. The internal oblique on the lower side of the body draws the upper-side shoulder toward the lower-side hip. The external and internal obliques on the upper side of the body combine to flex and laterally rotate the torso. Get a feel for this action in the preparatory pose with the feet still on the floor. Contract the abdomen in this position to isolate the oblique muscles alternately on each side of the body, and use them to increase the twist. These muscles stabilize the spine. Engage them in the final pose.

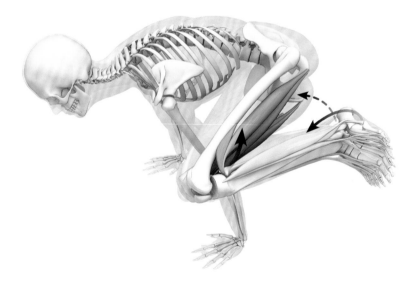

STEP 5 Flex the knees to squeeze the lower legs against the thighs, activating the hamstrings. Contract the tibialis anterior to dorsiflex the ankles. Extend the toes by engaging the extensors hallucis and digitorum. Evert the ankles to open the soles of the feet using the peronei. Balance this by co-activating the tibialis posterior muscles to augment the arches of the feet and create an inversion force at the ankle joints. This counters the eversion created by the peronei and stabilizes the ankles and feet. Engage the adductor muscles along the inner thighs to squeeze the knees together, locking them in place.

INVERSIONS

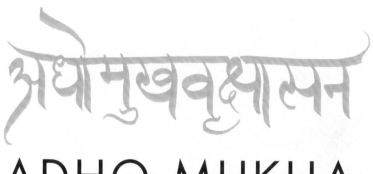

ADHO MUKHA VRKSASANA

FULL ARM BALANCE

ADHO MUKHA VRKSASANA IS AN INVERSION AS WELL AS AN ARM BALANCE. THE benefits of the inversion component include improved venous return to the heart with enhanced cardiac output and improved lymphatic flow into the thoracic duct.

We spend most of our lives in the bipedal position, walking, standing, etc. The hip joints are structured for weight-bearing in these types of activities. The shoulders, on the other hand, are highly mobile and designed for interacting with the environment through our hands. Practicing poses like Full Arm Balance reverses this design by turning the mobile shoulder joint into the joint that must be stable for weight-bearing. This strengthens the muscular stabilizers of the shoulder.

Stability and balance in this asana originate from the pelvis. In standing poses, we connect the feet with the pelvic core and then refine the pose via movements of the upper body. Here we connect the hands to the shoulder girdle and stabilize the pose from the pelvic core. Wobbling movement at the pelvis creates instability in the asana. This instability is transmitted to the upper extremities, where it is magnified, making it more work to hold the pose. Accordingly, stable arm balances require that the pelvic core muscles, such as the psoas and gluteals, are developed and awakened for yoga practice. Use the standing pose sequence provided in *Mat Companion 1* to awaken these core muscles.

BASIC JOINT POSITIONS

- The shoulders flex and externally rotate.
- The elbows extend.
- The forearms pronate.
- The wrists extend.
- The trunk extends.

- The hips extend and adduct.
- The knees extend.
- The ankles are neutral or plantar flex slightly.
- The feet evert.
- The toes extend.

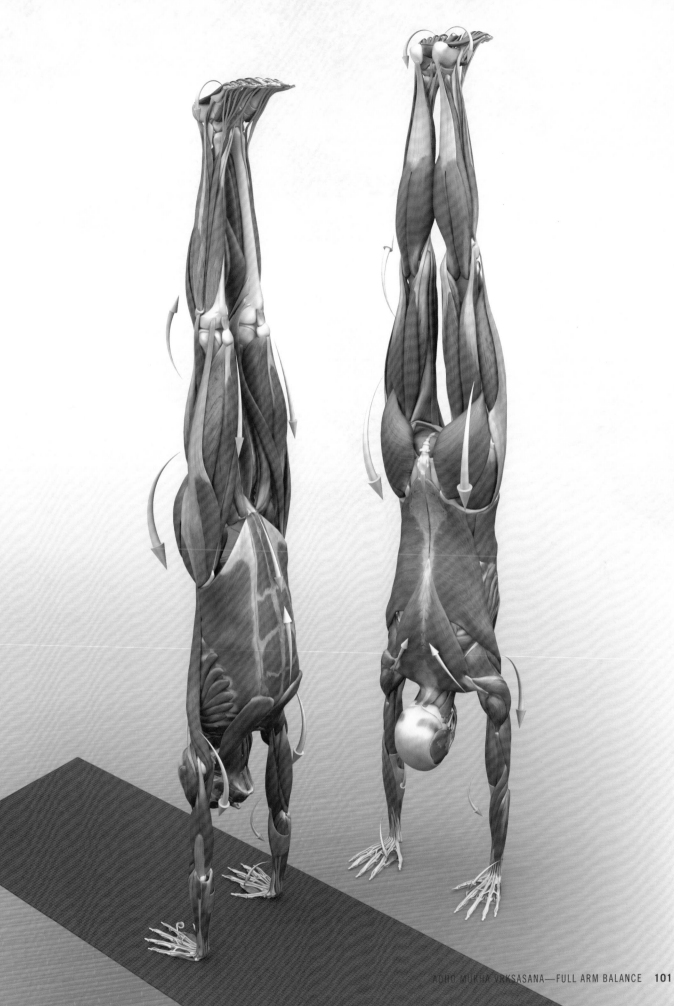

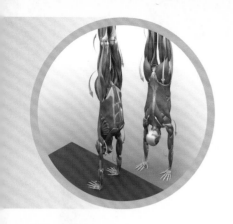

Adho Mukha Vrksasana Preparation

The act of going up into Full Arm Balance combines elements of physics and biomechanics. Joint rhythm couples with momentum, so that the body floats up into the pose with control.

Begin in Downward Facing Dog Pose. Then step one foot forward, keeping the knee bent. This shifts the center of gravity and brings the weight forward into the hands, taking the arms into a more vertical position. Pause here if you are new to the pose. Get used to positioning the arm bones so that the mechanical and anatomical axes align with one another.

Start to rock the weight over the hands in a 1-2-3 type of rhythm; then engage the thigh, buttocks, and lower back muscles to lift the back leg straight up onto the wall. Combine the momentum generated by rocking forward and back with the force of the spinal extensor muscles to lift the other leg.

Practice Dog Pose and Chaturanga Dandasana to gain strength in the shoulder girdle. Use Hanumanasana or its preparatory poses, as well as Warrior I, to gain flexibility and strength in the hips.

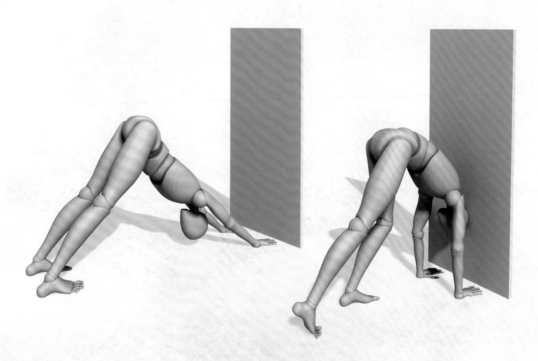

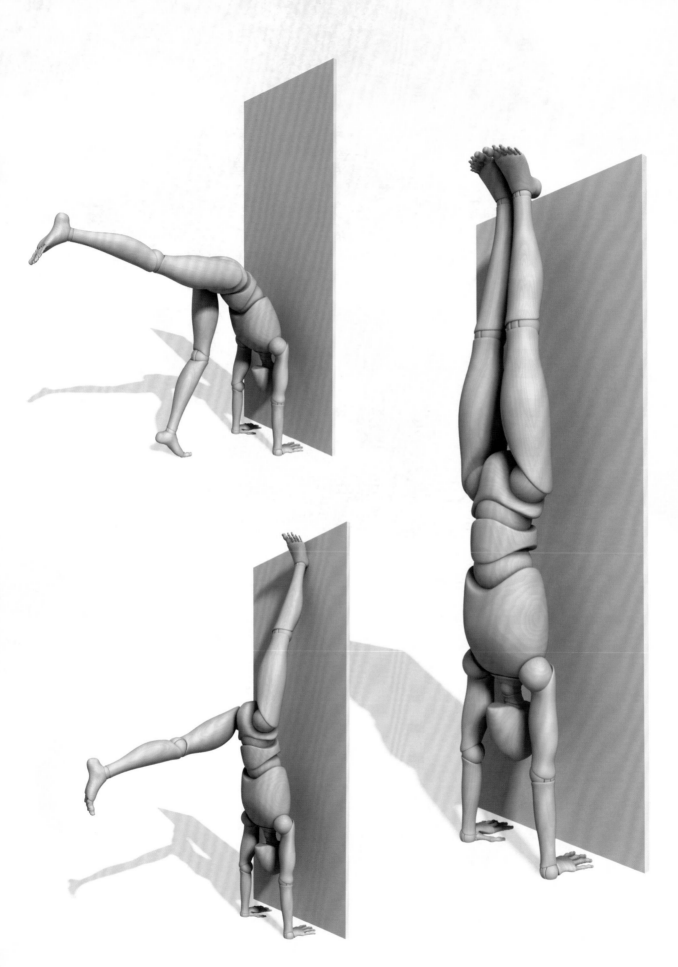

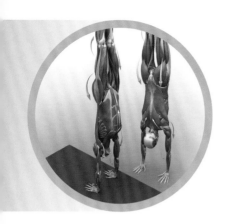

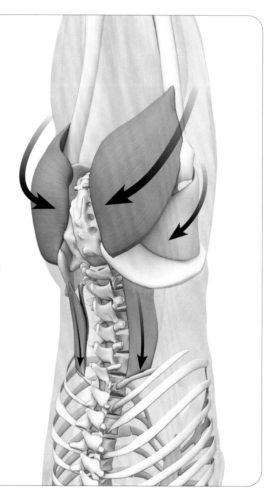

STEP 1 Engage the gluteus maximus to lift the leg into the air and create extension in the hip. Remember that the hip and pelvis move in rhythm and are connected to the lumbar spine. Activate the quadratus lumborum of the lower back. Notice how this draws the pelvis upward. Visualize the gluteus minimus contracting, deep in the side of the pelvis. When the hip is in a neutral position, this muscle stabilizes the head of the femur in the hip socket.

STEP 2 Activate the quadratus lumborum and erector spinae to extend the entire back into the pose. Ultimately you want the vertebral bodies to align one on top of the other, so that the force of gravity is balanced by the inherent flexibility of the intervertebral discs. The facet joints between each vertebra combine to stabilize the spine.

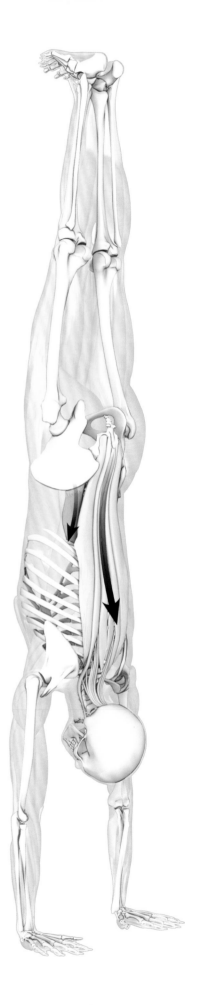

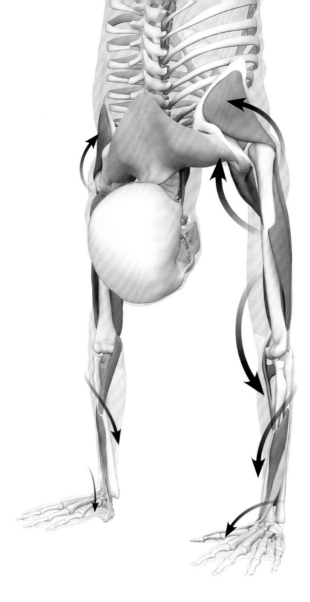

STEP 3 Use the arches of the palms to create a "spring" in the hands by gently flexing the fingers. Spread the fingers evenly and pronate the forearms by engaging the pronators teres and quadratus. This brings the weight into the mounds at the base of the index fingers. Then activate the infraspinatus and teres minor muscles to externally rotate the shoulders and shift the weight evenly across the hands. Note how pronating the forearms and externally rotating the shoulders creates a "coiling" force through the elbows. This tightens the elbow ligaments (ligamentotaxis) and stabilizes the arms. Counterbalance this action by spreading the weight evenly across the palms of the hands. This engages the supinator muscles of the forearms.

Link the shoulders to the hands by contracting the triceps to straighten the elbows. The long head of the triceps originates from the scapula, so engaging this muscle rotates the lower border of the scapula outward, drawing the acromion process away from the humerus, which allows greater forward flexion of the shoulder. Externally rotating the shoulder draws the greater tuberosity of the humerus away from the acromion. Accordingly, extending the elbows and externally rotating the shoulders frees the humeri to lift over the head without bony impingement. Contract the anterior deltoids to flex the shoulders overhead. Activate the upper third of the trapezius and the levator scapulae to elevate the shoulder girdle. Once in the pose, draw the shoulders away from the ears to free the neck.

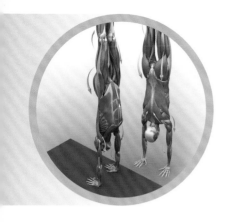

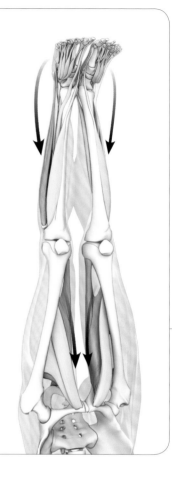

STEP 4 Squeeze the legs together to engage the adductor group of muscles on the inner thighs and stabilize the pelvis. Extend the toes with the long and short toe extensors. Activate the tibialis anterior muscle at the fronts of the lower legs to dorsiflex the ankles, bringing the soles of the feet toward parallel to the floor. Evert the ankles by contracting the peronei on the outsides of the lower legs, and then engage the tibialis posterior muscles to balance this with an inversion force. These co-activations stabilize the bones of the lower legs, ankles, and feet.

Opening the soles of the feet relieves tension and stimulates the minor chakras located in this region.

STEP 5 Contract the quadriceps to straighten the knees. A cue for this is to lift the kneecaps toward the pelvis. In Step 1 we engaged the gluteus maximus to extend the hip and lift the leg. This also causes some external rotation of the thigh. However, we want the femurs to be in a neutral position, with the kneecaps facing forward. Use the tensor fascia lata to counteract the external rotation and assist the quadriceps in straightening the knees. A cue for this is to imagine pressing the outer edges of the feet against an immovable object. This activates the abductor muscles (the tensor fascia lata and gluteus medius), which are also internal rotators of the hips. The legs are held together by the adductor group, but the thighs turn inward with this action and bring the kneecaps back to neutral.

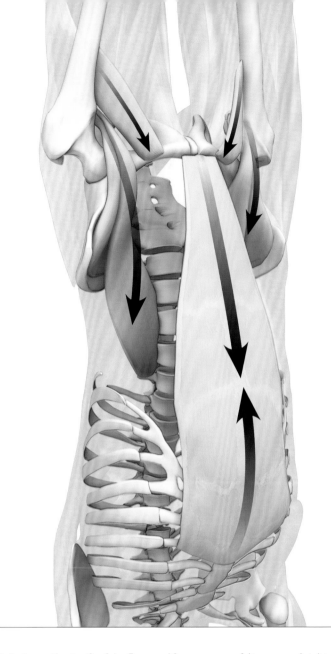

STEP 6 Co-activate the hip flexors (the psoas and its synergists) to balance the action of the hip extensors (the gluteus maximus and its synergists). This creates stability in the pose. You can gain awareness of this action by tilting the thighs slightly forward and back, refining the balance. Use the Psoas Awakening Series (see *The Key Poses of Yoga*) to obtain awareness and control of these core pelvic muscles.

Balance extension of the back with gentle activation of the abdominals. Note the attachment of the rectus abdominis on the front of the pelvis. Engaging this muscle creates a pull that counters the forward tilt of the pelvis, increasing stability.

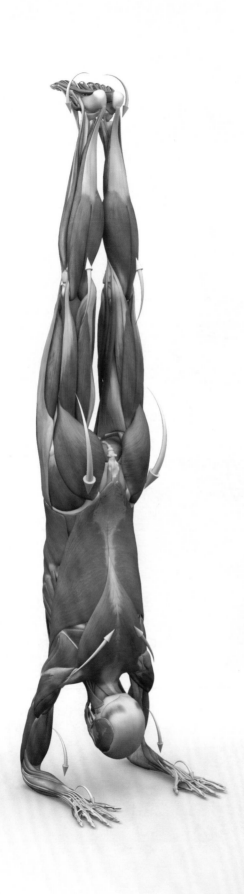
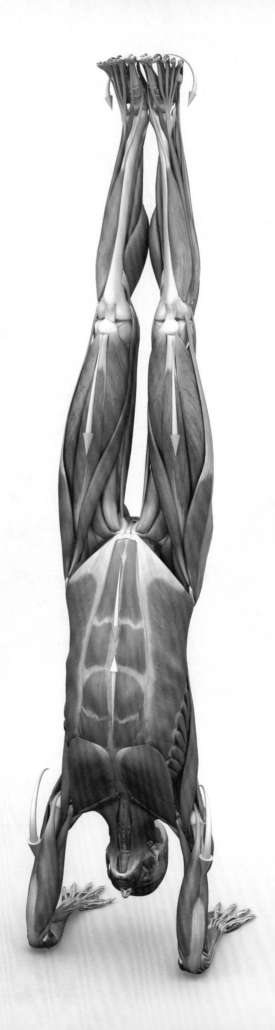

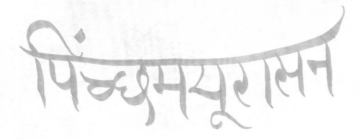

PINCHA MAYURASANA

FEATHERED PEACOCK POSE

IN PINCHA MAYURASANA THE WEIGHT OF THE BODY IS SPREAD ACROSS THE FOREARMS and into the palms. This pose shares the same benefits as Full Arm Balance, with the additional advantage of an unusual shoulder stretch. When the arms are held overhead in this position, the humeri are required to externally rotate near their maximum. This stretches the internal rotators of the shoulders. Tight internal rotators cause the hands to slide inward. Counter this tendency by preparing the shoulders with stretches such as Gomukhasana and Garudasana arms prior to taking the pose.

Remember that the shoulder is actually a combination of several joints. Use this knowledge to strategize how to obtain the optimal position of the pose. For example, protract the shoulder blades (move them away from the midline of the spine) to allow the elbows to adduct, or move inward. Protracting the scapulae also externally rotates the shoulders, but from the scapulothoracic joint rather than the shoulder joint proper. This allows the external rotators to more efficiently turn the humerus at the glenohumeral joint. Fix the shoulders in this position by pressing the hands into the mat. Then draw the scapulae back toward the midline of the spine. This is an example of using coupled joint actions to bring the body safely into a pose.

BASIC JOINT POSITIONS

- The shoulders flex and externally rotate.
- The elbows flex.
- The forearms pronate.
- The wrists flex.
- The trunk extends.
- The hips extend and adduct.

- The knees extend.
- The ankles are neutral or plantar flex slightly.
- The feet evert.
- The toes extend.
- The cervical spine extends.

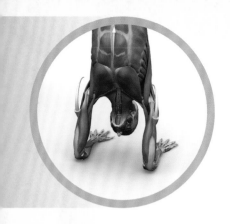

Pincha Mayurasana Preparation

Start on all fours with the forearms on the mat; then lift the knees. In the beginning, you can place a block between the hands and a belt around the elbows to position the forearms. Use Garudasana arms as well as the chair stretch illustrated below to prepare the shoulders. Work toward doing the pose without props.

Walk one foot forward to shift the weight and center of gravity over the shoulders and forearms. Then engage the muscles of the buttocks and lower back to lift the back leg. Keep one knee bent and the other straight and use momentum to bring the straight leg up onto the wall. Follow with the other leg. Then take one leg at a time away from the wall to learn to balance in this pose.

Use related postures such as Downward Facing Dog Pose, Chaturanga Dandasana, and Full Arm Balance to prepare for Pincha Mayurasana.

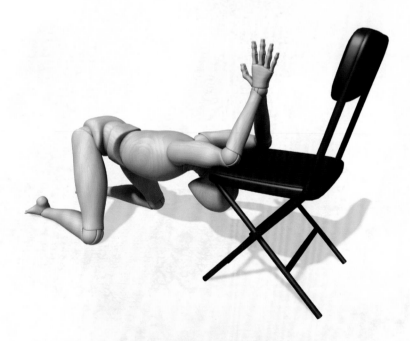

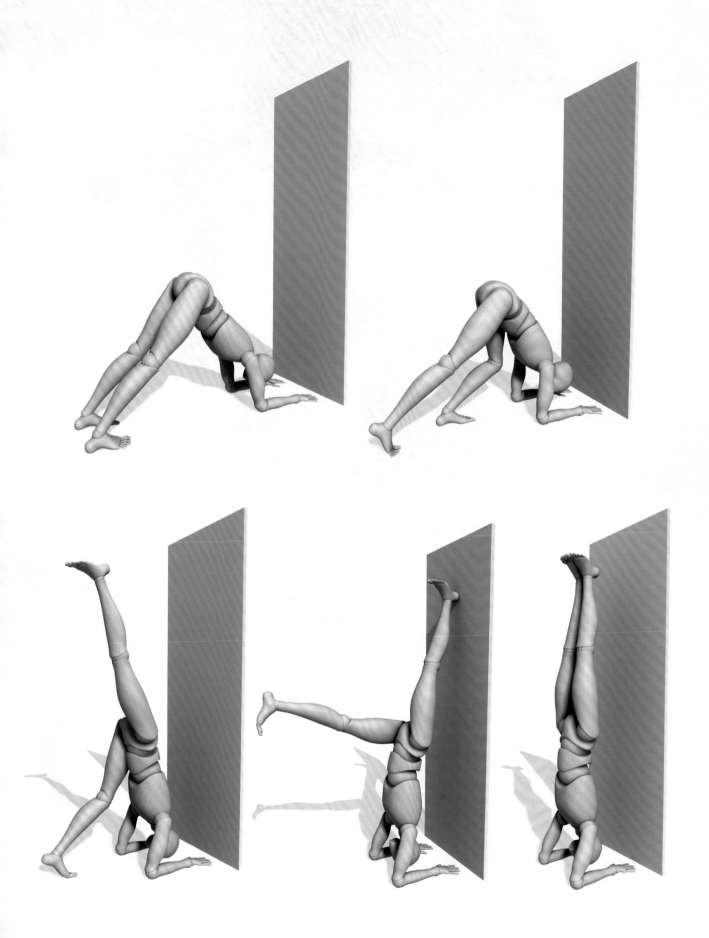

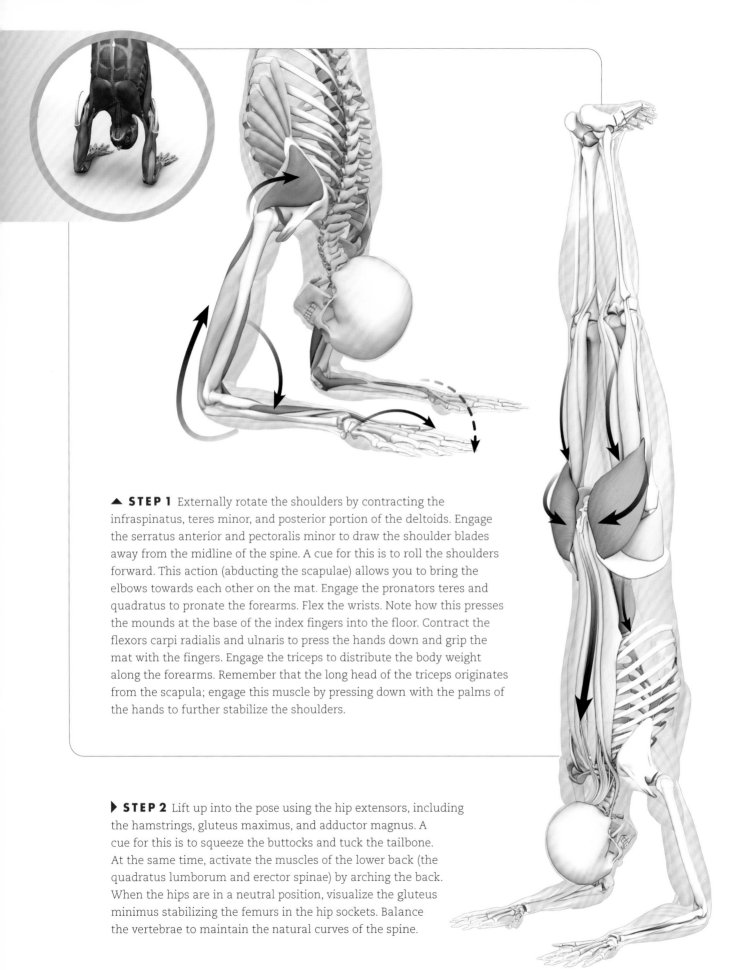

▲ **STEP 1** Externally rotate the shoulders by contracting the infraspinatus, teres minor, and posterior portion of the deltoids. Engage the serratus anterior and pectoralis minor to draw the shoulder blades away from the midline of the spine. A cue for this is to roll the shoulders forward. This action (abducting the scapulae) allows you to bring the elbows towards each other on the mat. Engage the pronators teres and quadratus to pronate the forearms. Flex the wrists. Note how this presses the mounds at the base of the index fingers into the floor. Contract the flexors carpi radialis and ulnaris to press the hands down and grip the mat with the fingers. Engage the triceps to distribute the body weight along the forearms. Remember that the long head of the triceps originates from the scapula; engage this muscle by pressing down with the palms of the hands to further stabilize the shoulders.

▶ **STEP 2** Lift up into the pose using the hip extensors, including the hamstrings, gluteus maximus, and adductor magnus. A cue for this is to squeeze the buttocks and tuck the tailbone. At the same time, activate the muscles of the lower back (the quadratus lumborum and erector spinae) by arching the back. When the hips are in a neutral position, visualize the gluteus minimus stabilizing the femurs in the hip sockets. Balance the vertebrae to maintain the natural curves of the spine.

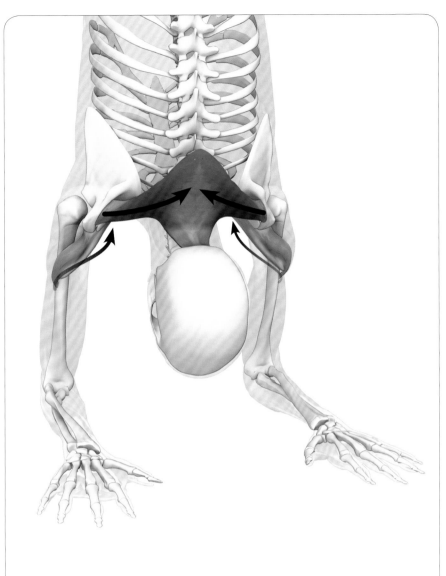

STEP 3 Lift the body upward from the shoulders by pressing down into the mat. This engages the levator scapulae, the upper third of the trapezius, and the serratus anterior. Contract these muscles in concert with those listed in Step 1.

STEP 4 Activate the quadriceps to straighten the knees. The tensor fascia lata synergizes the quadriceps in this action and internally rotates the thighs to a neutral position, so that the kneecaps face forward. Use the long and short toe extensors to extend the toes and dynamize the arches of the feet. Activate the tibialis anterior muscles at the fronts of the lower legs to dorsiflex the ankles, and evert the ankles using the peroneus longus and brevis to open the soles. Finally, engage the tibialis posterior muscles to create a slight inversion force at the ankle joints, stabilizing them.

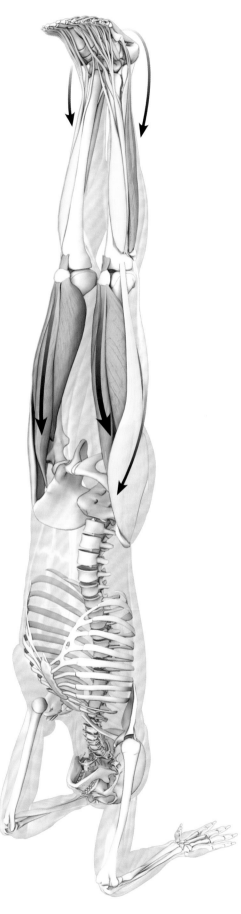

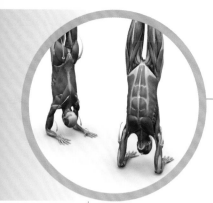

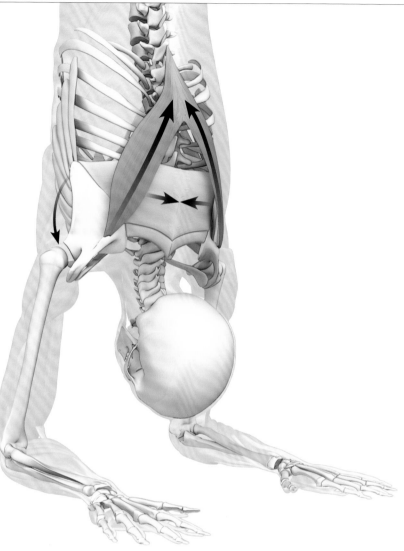

STEP 5 In Step 3 we use the shoulders to lift the body. In the final pose, however, we do not want to shrug the shoulders up against the neck. To avoid this, contract the lower trapezius and draw the scapulae away from the neck and ears. Attempt to draw the shoulder blades toward the midline by engaging the rhomboids, and then expand the chest outward by contracting the serratus anterior.

STEP 6 Activate the psoas and its synergists, the pectineus and adductors longus and brevis, to stabilize the pelvis. Squeezing the knees together is a cue for this action. These muscles prevent the torso and legs from swaying back over the arms. Engage the abdominals to stabilize the pelvis and protect the lumbar spine through the abdominal "air bag" effect.

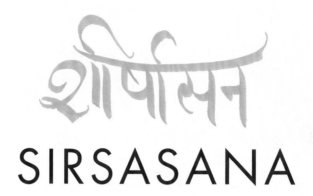

SIRSASANA

HEADSTAND

WE SPEND MOST OF OUR WAKING HOURS EITHER SITTING OR STANDING, WITH THE head above the heart. Headstand inverts and balances this habitual position, potentially affecting a variety of physiological processes. For example, there is an increase in the blood returning to the heart (venous return), which can improve (at least temporarily) cardiac output. Also, baroreceptors in the aorta and carotid arteries are stimulated, resulting in increased parasympathetic outflow from the central nervous system. This can, in turn, temporarily lower heart rate and blood pressure. Additionally, the cerebral spinal fluid that bathes the brain is likely affected, altering the flow to various regions and potentially improving the transport of nutrients to the brain. Headstand can also have musculoskeletal benefits, including strengthened paraspinous muscles and improved alignment of the vertebral column.

When you're in the pose, it is important to align the direction of the force of gravity with the anatomical axis of the vertebral column, such that the weight of the body is taken into the shoulders and distributed evenly throughout the intervertebral discs and vertebral bodies. The preparatory section below provides guidance on how to strengthen and train "muscle memory" in the paraspinous muscles, prior to actually going up into the pose.

Note, however, that Headstand can also be potentially hazardous, especially if you have any pathology in the cervical spine region. It should always be practiced under the direct supervision of a qualified instructor. If you choose not to practice Sirsasana, there are effective alternatives in the restorative pose sequence that allow you to obtain many of the benefits of inversions while avoiding the dangers.

BASIC JOINT POSITIONS

- The shoulders flex and externally rotate.
- The elbows flex.
- The forearms are neutral.
- The wrists flex.
- The trunk extends.
- The hips extend and adduct.
- The knees extend.
- The ankles are neutral or plantar flex slightly.
- The feet evert.
- The toes extend.

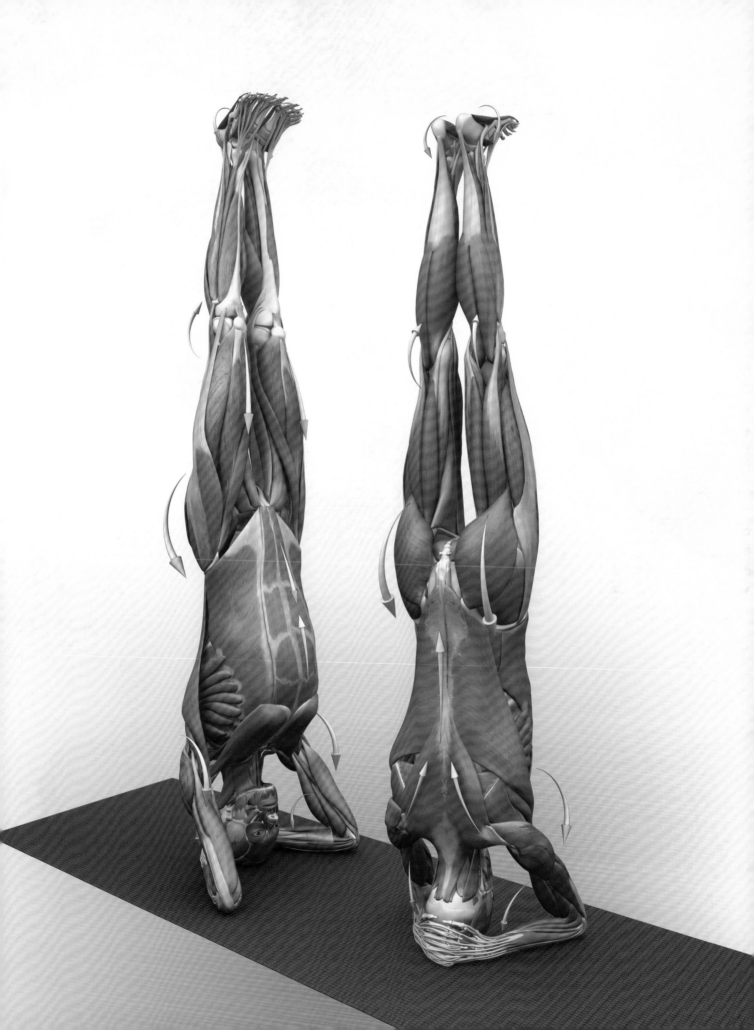

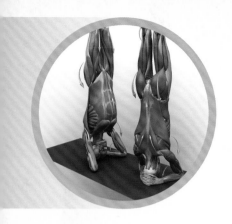

Sirsasana Preparation

Begin by strengthening and training the paraspinous muscles surrounding the vertebral column. Sit with the legs crossed, and align the vertebrae so that they "perch" directly over the pelvis. (See Easy Cross-Legged Pose in *Mat Companion 2* for details on this asana). Then place the palms of the hands on top of the head, as shown. Gently press onto the region of the fontanel, directly in the center of the skull. At the same time, press upward into the hands with the head. Initiate this effort from the pelvis and up through the aligned column. Hold this position for two to three breaths, and then rest the hands on the knees. Notice the lightness in the spine. Repeat once or twice.

Next, place the same fontanel region of the skull onto the mat between the interlocked hands. Keep most of the weight on the forearms and shoulders, and get a sense for pressing the top of the head gently into the mat. Hold this position for two or three breaths and then come out. Repeat once or twice, each time adding a little more weight onto the head to strengthen the paraspinous muscles while keeping most of the weight on the forearms and shoulders.

Use a wall for support in the beginning. Place the forearms and head in the same position on the floor. Draw the knees toward the chest and then bring the feet onto the wall, lifting up from the forearms and shoulders. Align the pelvis and shoulders. Hold this position for a few breaths and then come down into Child's Pose. Repeat this sequence. When you are ready, straighten the knees and extend into the final pose. If you have neck pain or numbness in the hands or arms, come out of the inversion and stop.

Remember that you should condition the paraspinous muscles over time. Work with the seated preparation and the intermediate Headstand shown here until you develop the strength to go up into full Sirsasana. Do not stand up immediately after doing Headstand or other inversions, as this can cause light-headedness. Always use an intermediary asana such as Child's Pose or Uttanasana to re-acclimate the cardiovascular system before standing straight up.

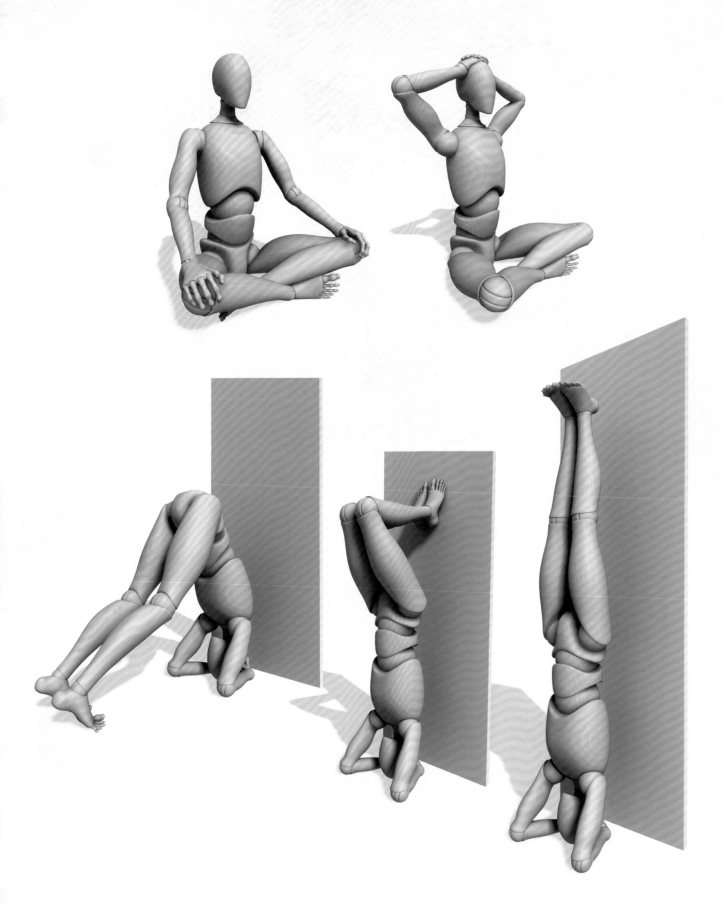

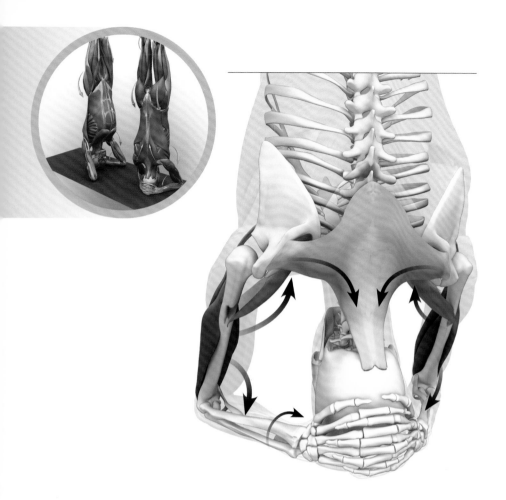

STEP 1 Align the shoulders and spine. Initially, press down through the shoulders by engaging the upper third of the trapezius. We will relax this muscle and draw the shoulders away from the ears as we progress in the pose. Contract the anterior portion of the deltoids as if raising the arms in front of you. Then engage the triceps and attempt to straighten the elbows; this presses the forearms into the mat. Pronate the forearms to squeeze the mounds at the base of the index fingers into the skull. We will balance this in Step 2 by co-activating the forearm supinators to maintain the wrists in a neutral position.

STEP 2 Use the biceps and brachialis muscles to counter the action of the triceps described in Step 1. In this pose, the action of the triceps predominates, with the biceps and brachialis muscles playing a stabilizing role. Flexing the elbows also brings the shoulders in line with the cervical spine and maintains the center of gravity over the head. This is necessary because pressing too hard onto the forearms (by contracting the triceps) can shift the body weight over the elbows. Shifting the weight over the elbows potentially causes problems because there is a tendency to counter this by contracting the extensor muscles of the neck to hold the body up.

Engage the biceps and supinator muscles to counterbalance the action of the forearm pronators (Step 1) by pressing the little finger sides of the palms into the skull. In this way, the wrists remain in a neutral position.

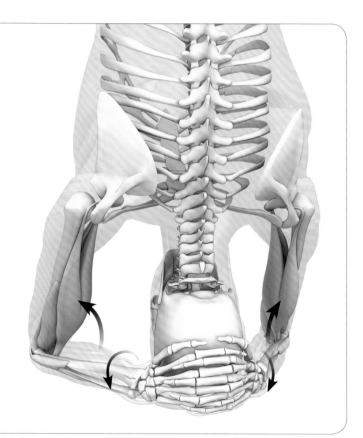

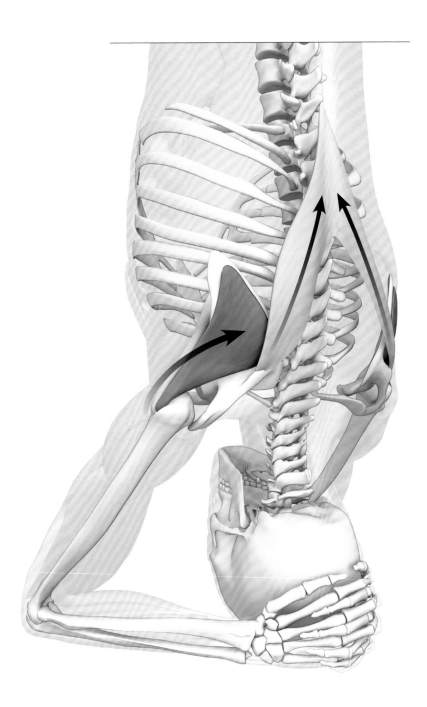

STEP 3 Externally rotate the upper arm bones (the humeri) by contracting the infraspinatus and teres minor muscles of the rotator cuff. This stabilizes the head of the humerus in the socket. Contract the lower third of the trapezius to draw the shoulders away from the ears, freeing the cervical spine.

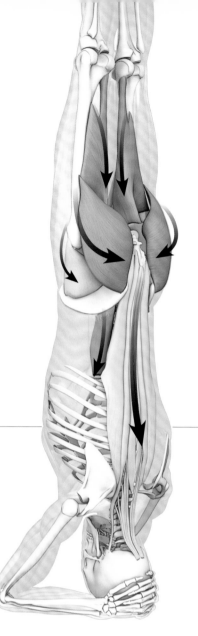

◄ STEP 4 Combine the actions of the gluteus maximus and adductor magnus to extend the hips in the pose. The cue for this is to gently squeeze the buttocks while drawing the knees together. Visualize the gluteus minimus stabilizing the head of the femur in the socket (this is its action when the femur is in neutral, as in Headstand). Use the erector spinae and quadratus lumborum to slightly arch the back. You will counter and stabilize this action in Step 5 by engaging the rectus abdominis and psoas muscles.

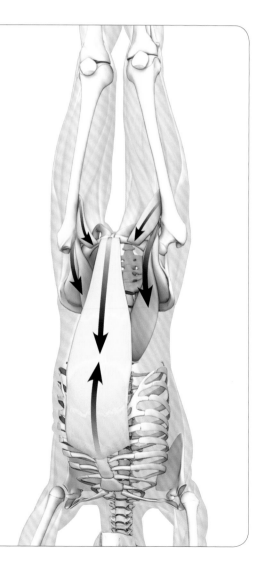

► STEP 5 Activating the gluteus maximus too strongly can result in a "swayback" posture. Engage the psoas and pectineus muscles at the front of the pelvis to bring the thighs back to a neutral position. Firm the abdomen by gently contracting the rectus abdominis. This counters overarching in the region of the lumbar spine.

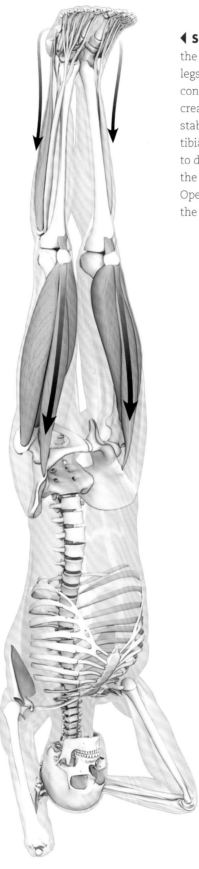

◀ **STEP 7** Evert the ankles by engaging the peronei at the sides of the lower legs. Then balance this action by contracting the tibialis posterior to create an inversion force at the ankles, stabilizing them. Finally, engage the tibialis anterior and the toe extensors to draw the tops of the feet toward the shins and open the soles upward. Opening the soles of the feet stimulates the minor chakras in this region.

▶ **STEP 6** Activate the quadriceps to straighten the knees. When we extend the hips by contracting the gluteus maximus, there is a tendency to externally rotate the thighs and turn the kneecaps to face outward. Engage the tensor fascia lata and gluteus medius to bring the thighs back to neutral. The cue for this is to imagine pressing the outer edges of the feet against an immovable object. This activates the abductor component of these muscles, which are also internal rotators of the hips. The legs do not pull apart; however, the external rotation is neutralized as the thighs turn inward and the kneecaps are brought to face forward. You can train this action by tying a belt snugly around the thighs and attempting to press the legs outward.

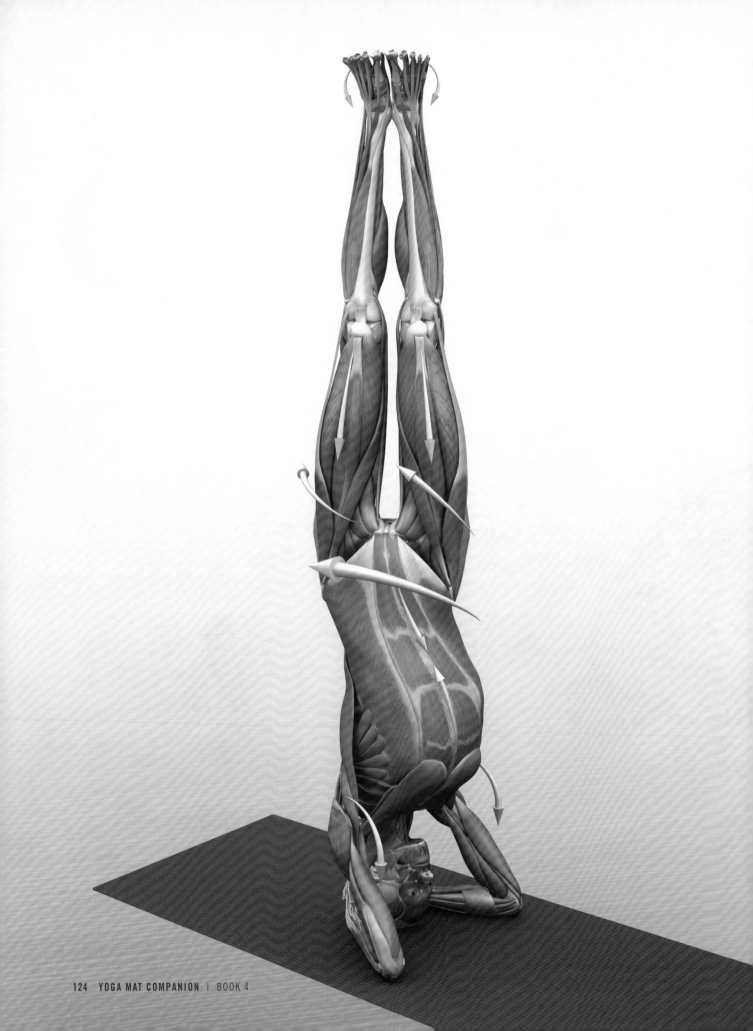

पार्श्वशीर्षासन

PARSVA SIRSASANA

REVOLVING HEADSTAND

PARSVA SIRSASANA IS THE TURNING VERSION OF HEADSTAND. IT HAS MANY OF the same potential benefits as the other inversions, including effects on the cardiovascular system (increased venous return, improved cardiac output, lowered heart rate and blood pressure) and a flushing effect on the cerebrospinal fluid. The coil created through the torso produces a kriya that augments the flushing of fluids through the detoxifying organs. These include the liver and spleen, as well as the lymphatics within the digestive system. Toxins are then directed from these organs into the major vessels of the cardiovascular system and eventually eliminated via the kidneys, lungs, and skin.

Like other twisting poses, Parsva Sirsasana involves turning the shoulder girdle in one direction and the pelvic girdle in the other. As in all inversions, the weight of the body in this pose is at least partially borne by the head and neck. It is dangerous to put a compressive force on the cervical spine while turning it, as this can place undue stress on the intervertebral discs and on the facet joints between the vertebral bodies. For this reason, the cervical spine should at all times have freedom of movement, a natural curvature, and minimal pressure on the head. Most of the body weight should be taken in the shoulders while keeping the neck relaxed.

It is essential to understand the biomechanics of the shoulder and pelvic girdles in order to obtain the greatest benefits from this pose. For example, when you turn the pelvic girdle, the force is transmitted through the torso, which tends to turn the shoulders in the same direction. This is a potentially dangerous situation that can result in tortional compression of the cervical spine, as described above. Use the shoulders to resist the turn so that the neck remains in a relaxed and neutral position. The steps below describe which muscles to engage to accomplish this.

BASIC JOINT POSITIONS

- The shoulders flex and externally rotate.
- The elbows flex.
- The forearms are neutral.
- The wrists flex.
- The trunk extends and rotates.

- The hips extend and adduct.
- The knees extend.
- The ankles are neutral or plantar flex slightly.
- The feet evert.
- The toes extend.

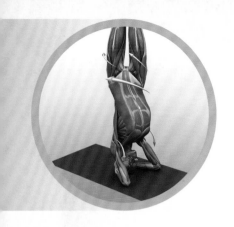

Parsva Sirsasana
Preparation

Use the preparatory steps described for Sirsasana (Headstand). You can prepare the torso for Revolving Headstand with the chair twist illustrated here. Practice near a wall in the beginning. Press down through the forearms to stabilize the base and take the weight off the cervical spine. Come up into Sirsasana.

Then turn the body so that the side of the hip and thigh remain on the wall. There will be a tendency for one shoulder to turn back while the other follows the same-side hip and turns forward. Resist this tendency using the steps described below. Keep the neck relaxed and neutral and return to Headstand. Carefully come down and rest in Child's Pose.

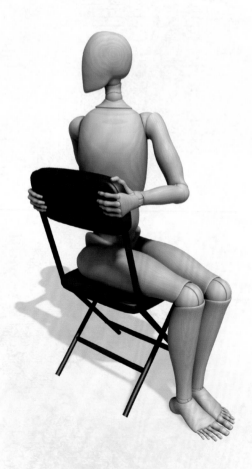

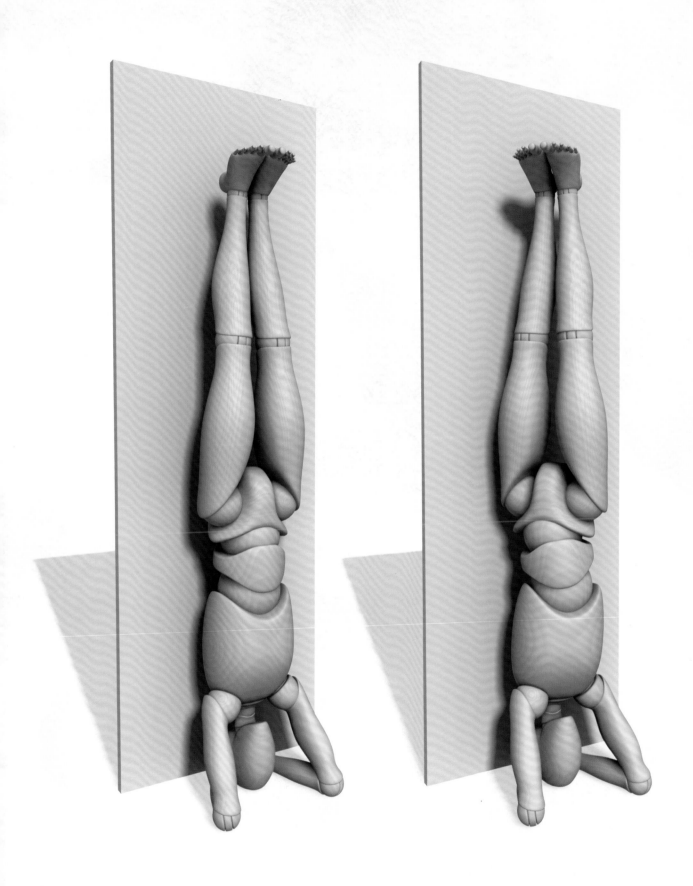

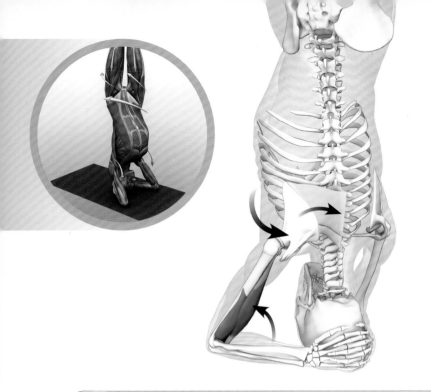

STEP 1 When you twist the lower body, the shoulder that you are twisting away from tends to move forward. Counter this by engaging the rhomboids major and minor to draw the scapula back and toward the midline. Flex the elbow by contracting the biceps and brachialis. Because the forearm is on the mat, the net effect of this action is to draw the shoulder back.

Squeeze the palms into the skull, mainly on the little finger side, by activating the supinator muscles of the forearms. The biceps synergizes this action. We will balance this movement of the forearms in Step 2.

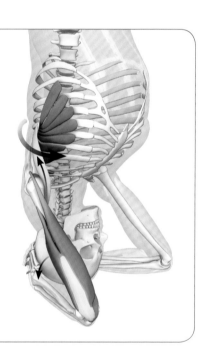

STEP 2 The shoulder on the side that you are twisting toward will tend to move back in the direction of the twist. Engage the serratus anterior to counter this tendency by pulling the shoulder blade forward. The teres major contributes to this action by drawing the edge of the scapula forward. Imagine pushing against a wall with the hand to get a feeling for bringing the shoulder blade back toward the front. Then press down onto the forearm by attempting to straighten the elbow. This activates the triceps.

Press the mounds at the base of the index fingers into the skull by contracting the pronator teres and quadratus muscles of the forearms. This pronation force balances the supination of the forearms described in Step 1 and stabilizes the wrists.

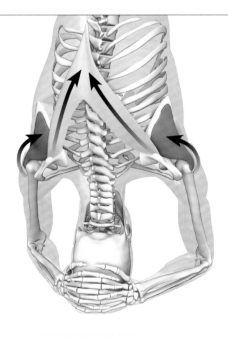

STEP 3 Externally rotate the upper arms by contracting the infraspinatus and teres minor muscles. The posterior third of the deltoids contributes to this action. Draw the shoulders away from the ears to free the neck. Engage the lower third of the trapezius to pull the shoulder girdle upward on the back, as shown.

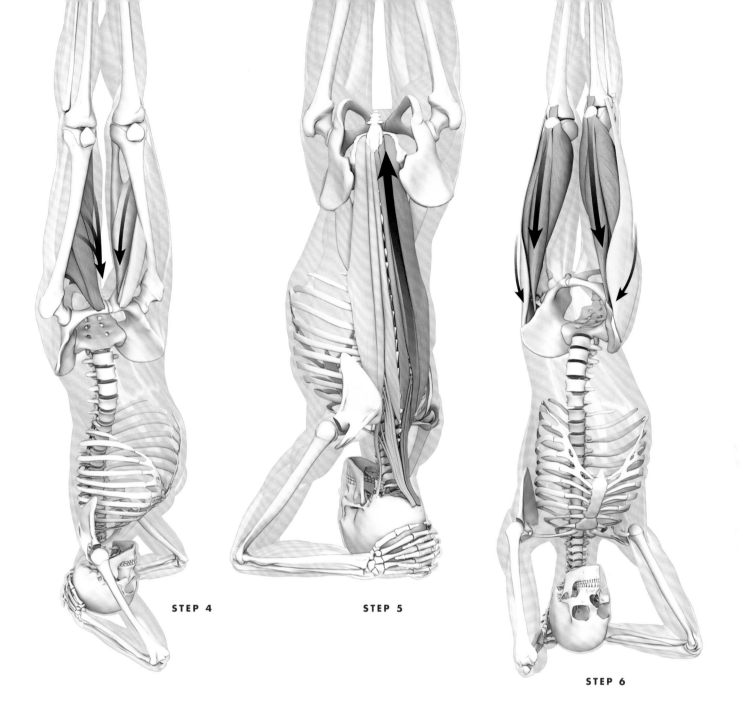

STEP 4   Contract the adductor group of muscles on the insides of the thighs. The cue for this is to squeeze the knees together. Engage the adductors more forcefully on the leg that leads the turn. This synergizes the twist of the lower body.

STEP 5   Contract the erector spinae and quadratus lumborum muscles to slightly arch the back on the side you are twisting toward, accentuating the turn of the body. The side of the back that is away from the twist stretches, as shown.

STEP 6   Activate the quadriceps to straighten the knees. The tensor fascia lata synergizes this action to stabilize the knee joint and, with the gluteus medius, internally rotates the thigh. The cue for contracting these muscles while in Headstand is to imagine pressing outward with the edges of the feet. The adductor group (in Step 4) prevents the legs from actually abducting out to the side; however, the effort to engage these muscles activates their internal rotation component and turns the thighs back toward neutral.

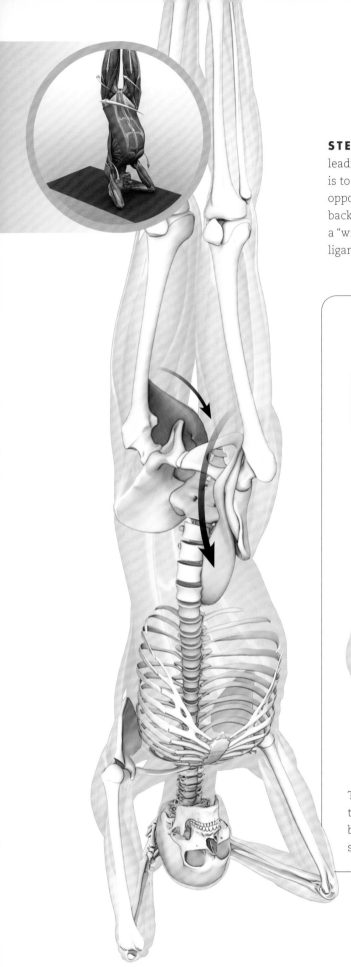

STEP 7 Engage the pelvic core. Contract the psoas on the side that is leading the twist to draw that side of the pelvis forward. The cue for this is to slightly flex the hips from the tops of the thighs. Then squeeze the opposite-side buttocks to activate the gluteus maximus by arching the back and tucking the tailbone under. Activating these muscles produces a "wringing," or "coiling," effect across the pelvis, tightening the sacroiliac ligaments. This stabilizes the entire pose and deepens the twist.

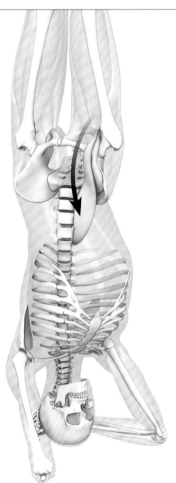

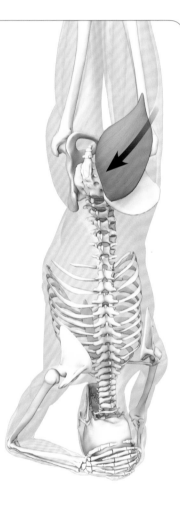

This is an isolated view of the pelvic bandha produced by engaging the psoas on the side that turns into the twist.

This is a back view demonstrating the other side of the bandha created by contracting the gluteus maximus.

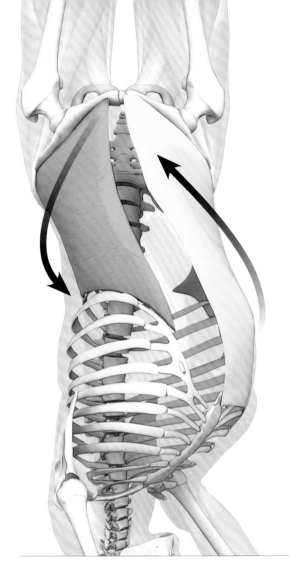

▲ **STEP 8** Move the twist down the body and into the trunk. Tighten the oblique abdominals to turn into the twist. In addition to turning the body, engaging these muscles raises intra-abdominal pressure, producing the "air bag" effect and stabilizing the lumbar spine.

▶ **SUMMARY** Parsva Sirsasana lengthens the spinal rotators and erector spinae, as well as the transversus abdominis and oblique abdominals.

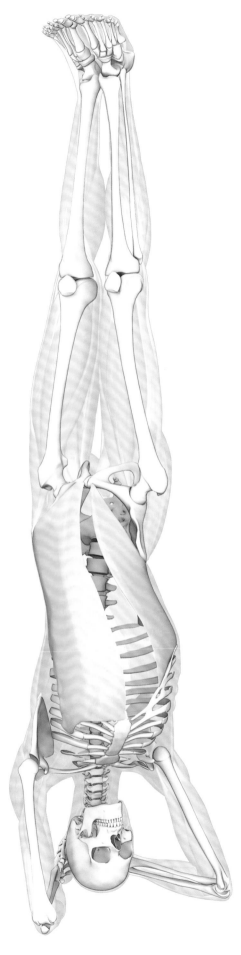

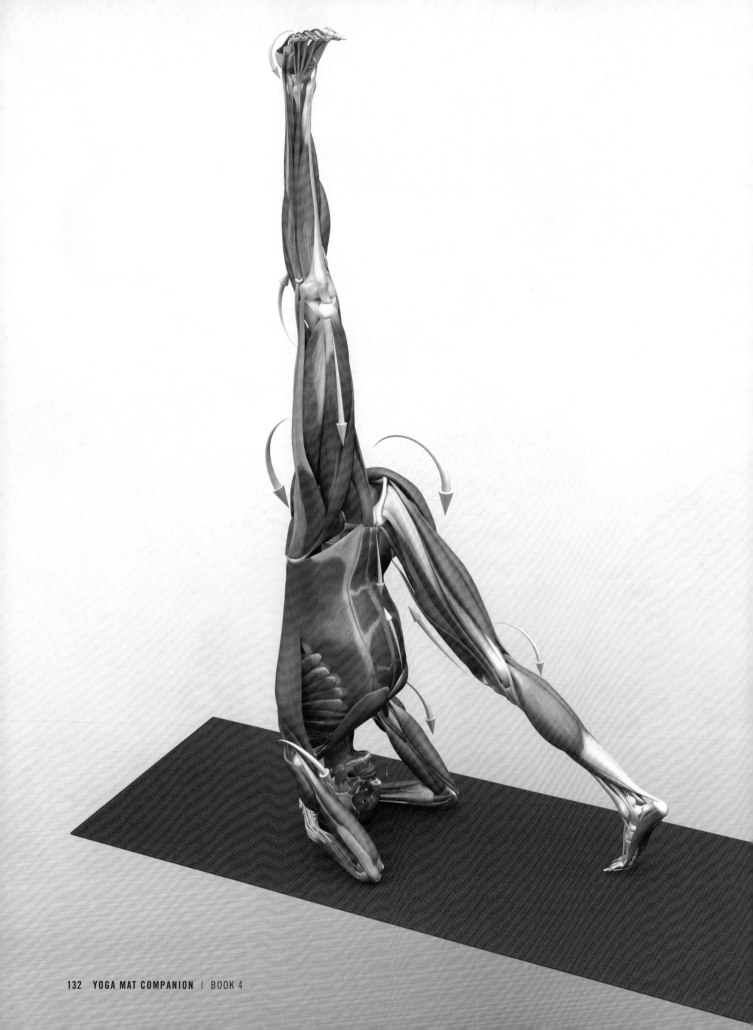

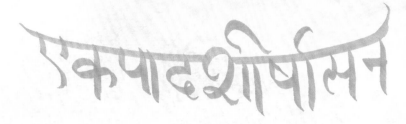

EKA PADA SIRSASANA

ONE-LEGGED HEADSTAND

EKA PADA SIRSASANA COMBINES AN INVERSION WITH A STRETCH OF THE gastrocnemius, hamstrings, and gluteals of the leg that is brought forward and down. This means there are three separate stories taking place in the pose: an inversion, a leg that is lowered to the ground, and a leg that remains in the air. The trunk is also important. There is a tendency to collapse the side of the body and the hip when lowering the leg. You can counter this by engaging the muscles on the other side of the trunk to expand the side that is shortening.

Combine the actions of the two legs by co-contracting the core muscles of the pelvis, including the psoas of the flexing hip and the gluteals of the leg that remains in the air. This creates a bandha across the pelvis, tightening the sacroiliac ligaments and stabilizing the pose.

Approach this head balance so that the weight of the body rebounds up through the vertebral column while preserving the natural spinal curves. Align the mechanical axis (the direction of gravity) with the anatomical axis of the spinal column. Avoid leaning forward by firmly engaging the gluteal and lower back muscles. Do not use the neck to attempt to draw the body forward, as this can cause injury. Instead, engage the muscles around the shoulder girdle, and press the sides of the forearms into the mat to support the body weight while keeping the neck free. Use the shoulders and arms to brace the body as you ease out of the pose.

BASIC JOINT POSITIONS

- The shoulders flex and externally rotate.
- The elbows flex.
- The forearms are neutral.
- The wrists flex.
- The trunk extends.
- The lifted-leg hip extends, adducts, and internally rotates.
- The lowered-leg hip flexes.
- The knees extend.
- The raised-leg ankle is neutral or plantar flexes slightly.
- The lowered-leg ankle dorsiflexes.
- The feet evert.
- The toes extend.

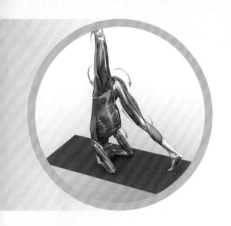

Eka Pada Sirsasana
Preparation

Prepare for Eka Pada Sirsasana with poses such as Parsvottanasana and Hanuma-nasana (or variations of these) to stretch the hamstrings, gluteals, and hip flexors. Use the Psoas Awakening Series (described in *The Key Poses of Yoga*) to gain conscious control of the core pelvic musculature, including the psoas and gluteals.

Begin with the same preparation used for Headstand. Once you are comfortable in Sirsasana, try variations such as Eka Pada Sirsasana. In the beginning, use the wall or a chair to support the foot in coming halfway down. Then lower the foot further and eventually bring it to the floor. Return to full Headstand before changing sides. Come out of the pose from Sirsasana; carefully lower both feet to the floor and rest in Child's Pose before standing up. This allows the cardiovascular system to re-acclimate.

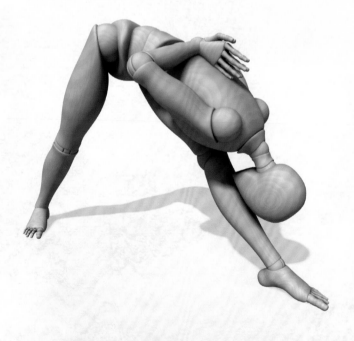

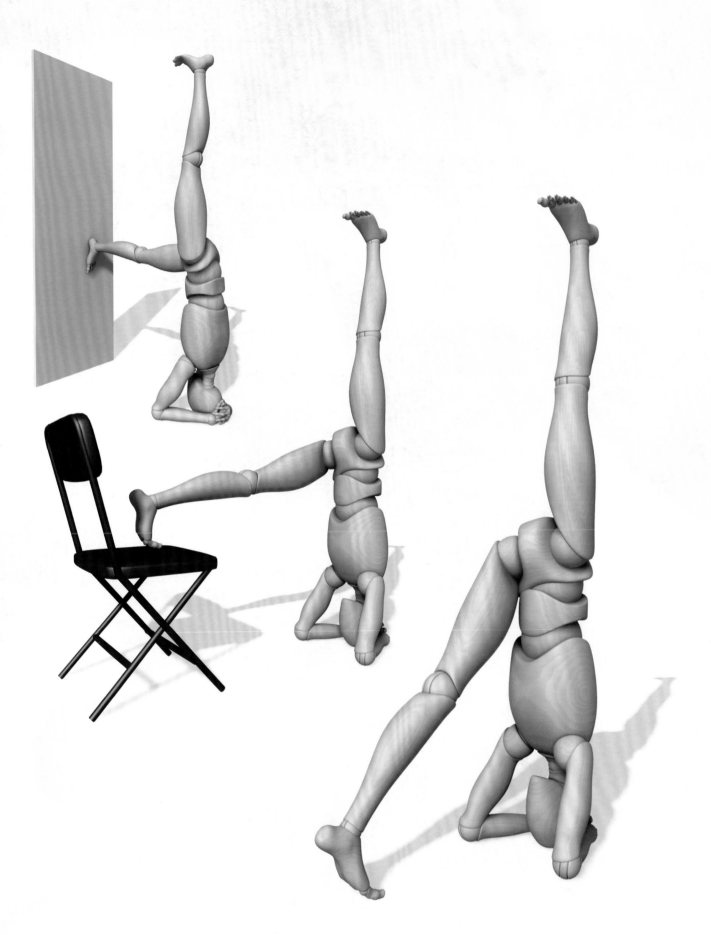

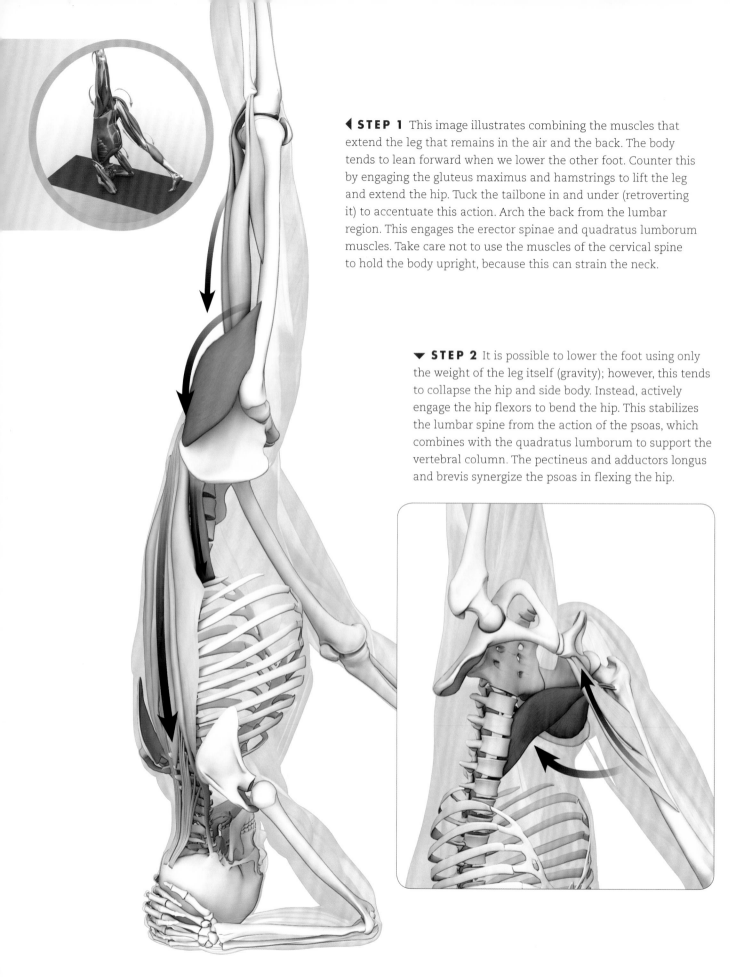

◀ STEP 1 This image illustrates combining the muscles that extend the leg that remains in the air and the back. The body tends to lean forward when we lower the other foot. Counter this by engaging the gluteus maximus and hamstrings to lift the leg and extend the hip. Tuck the tailbone in and under (retroverting it) to accentuate this action. Arch the back from the lumbar region. This engages the erector spinae and quadratus lumborum muscles. Take care not to use the muscles of the cervical spine to hold the body upright, because this can strain the neck.

▼ STEP 2 It is possible to lower the foot using only the weight of the leg itself (gravity); however, this tends to collapse the hip and side body. Instead, actively engage the hip flexors to bend the hip. This stabilizes the lumbar spine from the action of the psoas, which combines with the quadratus lumborum to support the vertebral column. The pectineus and adductors longus and brevis synergize the psoas in flexing the hip.

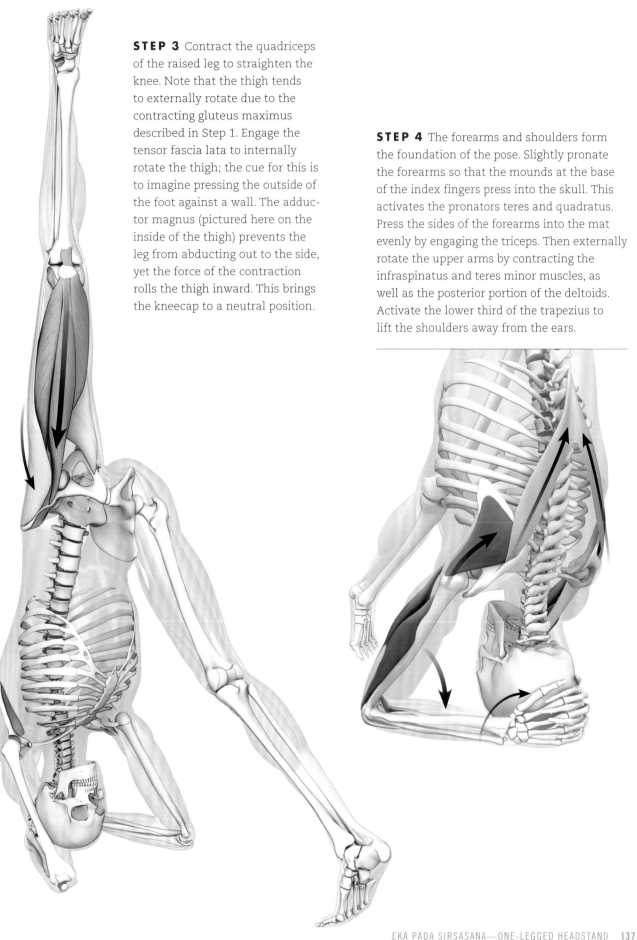

STEP 3 Contract the quadriceps of the raised leg to straighten the knee. Note that the thigh tends to externally rotate due to the contracting gluteus maximus described in Step 1. Engage the tensor fascia lata to internally rotate the thigh; the cue for this is to imagine pressing the outside of the foot against a wall. The adductor magnus (pictured here on the inside of the thigh) prevents the leg from abducting out to the side, yet the force of the contraction rolls the thigh inward. This brings the kneecap to a neutral position.

STEP 4 The forearms and shoulders form the foundation of the pose. Slightly pronate the forearms so that the mounds at the base of the index fingers press into the skull. This activates the pronators teres and quadratus. Press the sides of the forearms into the mat evenly by engaging the triceps. Then externally rotate the upper arms by contracting the infraspinatus and teres minor muscles, as well as the posterior portion of the deltoids. Activate the lower third of the trapezius to lift the shoulders away from the ears.

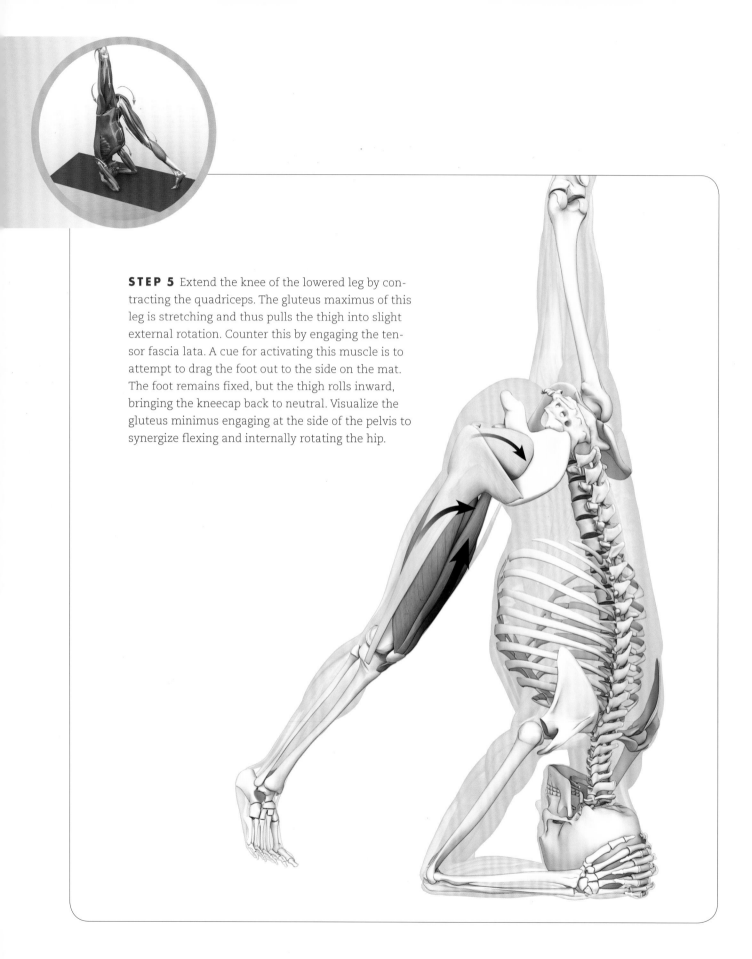

STEP 5 Extend the knee of the lowered leg by contracting the quadriceps. The gluteus maximus of this leg is stretching and thus pulls the thigh into slight external rotation. Counter this by engaging the tensor fascia lata. A cue for activating this muscle is to attempt to drag the foot out to the side on the mat. The foot remains fixed, but the thigh rolls inward, bringing the kneecap back to neutral. Visualize the gluteus minimus engaging at the side of the pelvis to synergize flexing and internally rotating the hip.

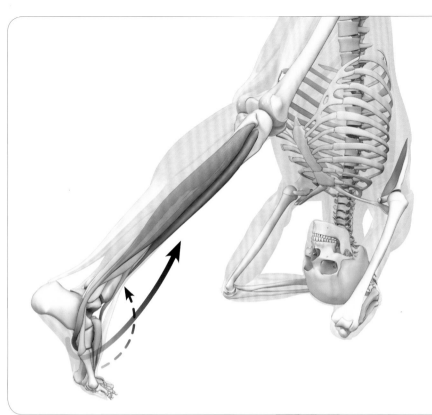

STEP 6 Activate the peroneus longus and brevis muscles to evert the ankle and the tibialis anterior to dorsiflex it (draw the top of the foot toward the shin). Engage the tibialis posterior to balance these actions and create a slight inversion force at the joint. This dynamizes the arch of the foot and stabilizes the ankle.

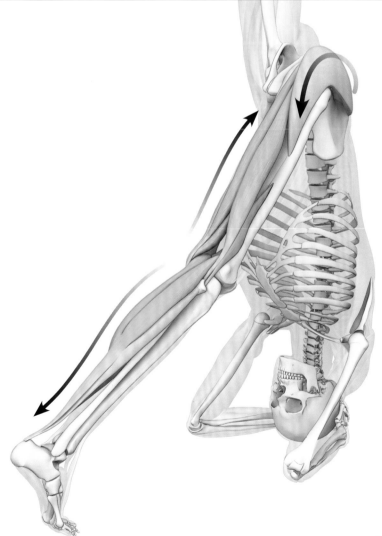

SUMMARY Eka Pada Sirsasana trains balance on a deeper level than classic Sirsasana. Become aware of how your Headstand with both legs in the air changes after you do this variation. Lowering the leg stretches the gastrocnemius/ soleus complex, hamstrings, and gluteus maximus. The erector spinae and quadratus lumborum on the lowered-leg side also lengthen.

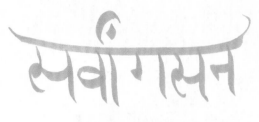

SALAMBA SARVANGASANA

SUPPORTED SHOULDER STAND

SALAMBA SARVANGASANA IS THE FIRST SHOULDER STAND INVERSION. WHERE Headstand has the shoulders flexing forward, Shoulder Stand has them extending, with the hands supporting the back. Additionally, the neck is flexed. As with other postures, there are several subplots to the story of Sarvangasana—an inversion, a shoulder stretch, and a chest opener. Do not place the weight of the body onto the neck. Instead, lean back into the hands and elbows to distribute the weight across the shoulders and upper arms. This frees the neck. At the same time, contract the biceps to press the hands into the back. This levers the chest open—one of the great hidden benefits of the pose. Shoulder Stand also shares many of the potential benefits of other inversions, including improved venous return and cardiac output and increased parasympathetic outflow (temporarily lowering heart rate and blood pressure).

BASIC JOINT POSITIONS

- The shoulders extend and externally rotate.
- The elbows flex.
- The forearms supinate.
- The trunk extends.
- The cervical spine flexes.

- The hips extend and adduct.
- The knees extend.
- The ankles are neutral or plantar flex slightly.
- The feet evert.
- The toes extend (the big toe can flex).

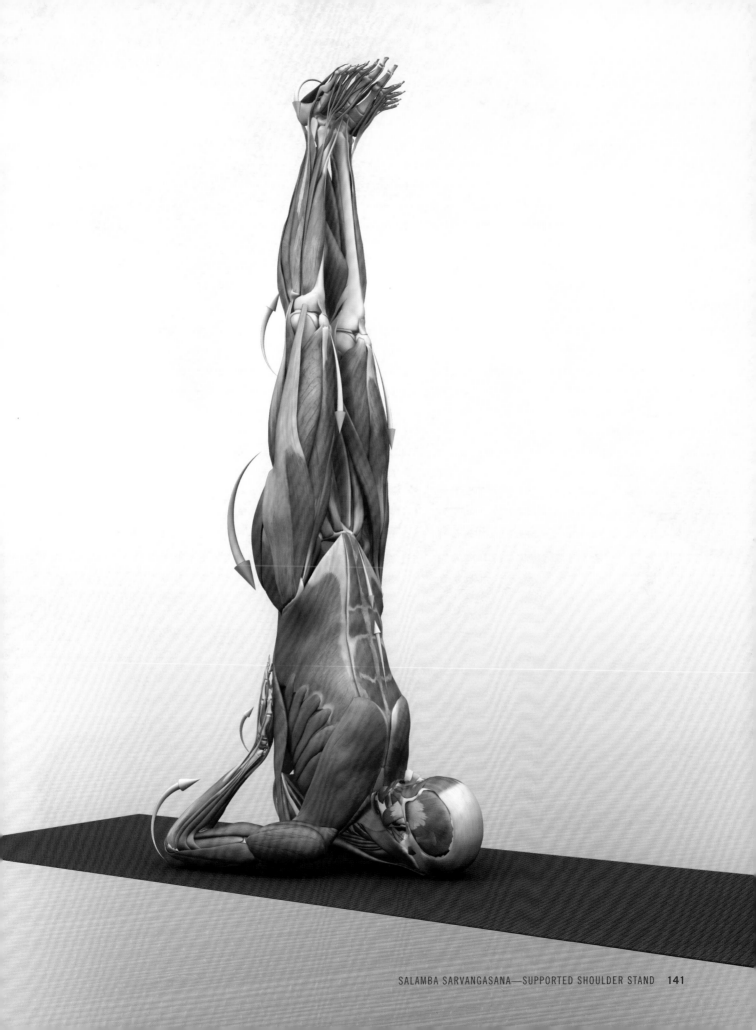

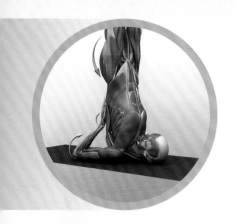

Salamba Sarvangasana
Preparation

Begin by stretching the shoulder flexors at the front of the chest and the arms by using the same facilitated stretches we used in Purvottanasana. Take care not to hyperextend the wrists in this preparation.

Try the supported variation of the pose by using a chair against a wall and a blanket or bolster under the shoulders. In the beginning, rest the feet against the wall and grasp the legs of the chair to open the chest. Then take the feet and legs straight up. These variations of Shoulder Stand can be combined with other restorative poses, such as Setu Bandha Sarvangasana and Viparita Karani.

As you progress to the free-standing variation, roll up from flat on the back or begin in Halasana and draw the knees into the chest; then come into the pose by extending the legs and leaning into the hands. You can also place a belt around the thighs to tether the legs together. Open the soles of the feet upwards by extending the toes and everting the ankles.

Brace the back with the hands to ease out of the pose. Roll onto the back and rest there for a few moments to allow the cardiovascular system to readjust.

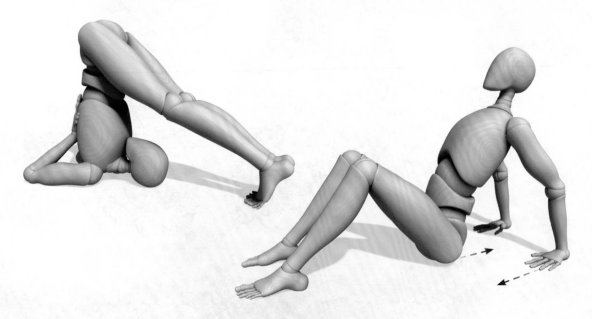

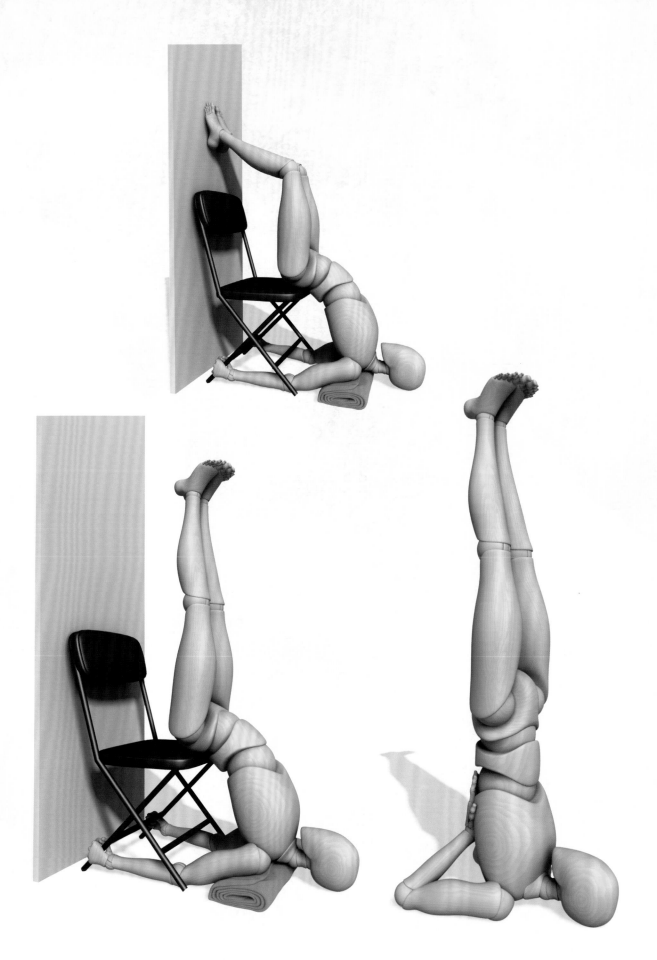

SALAMBA SARVANGASANA—SUPPORTED SHOULDER STAND **143**

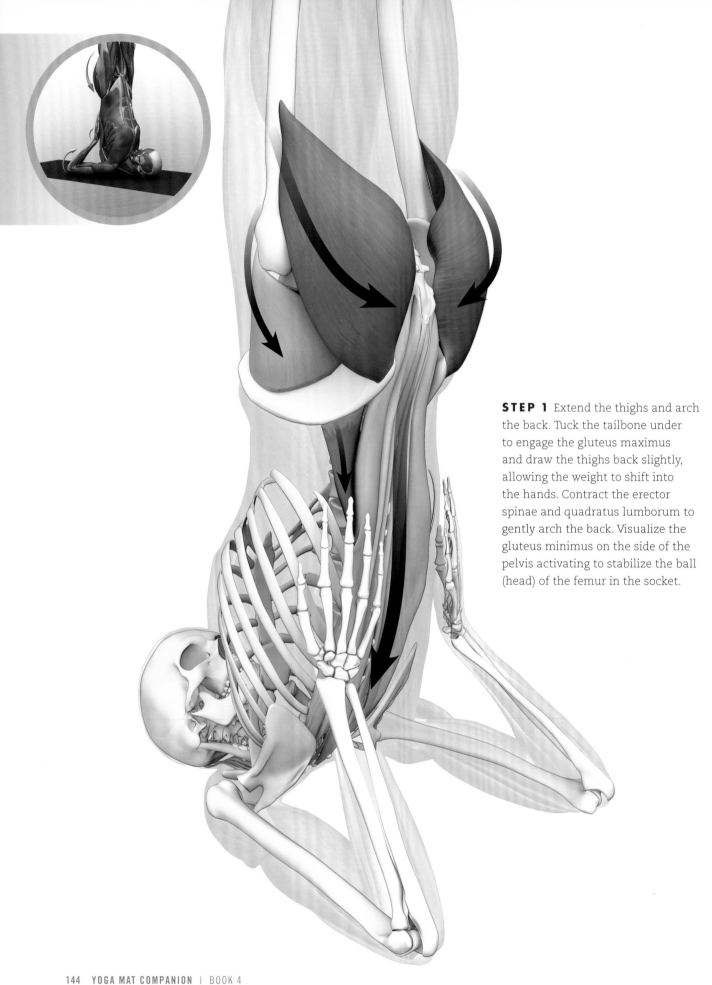

STEP 1 Extend the thighs and arch the back. Tuck the tailbone under to engage the gluteus maximus and draw the thighs back slightly, allowing the weight to shift into the hands. Contract the erector spinae and quadratus lumborum to gently arch the back. Visualize the gluteus minimus on the side of the pelvis activating to stabilize the ball (head) of the femur in the socket.

STEP 2 Flex the elbows to press the palms into the back. Lean into the hands and contract the biceps and brachialis muscles to support the weight and expand the chest forward. This is a key action in the pose. Press the backs of the arms into the mat by engaging the posterior deltoids. This aids to stretch the muscles at the front of the chest and produces reciprocal inhibition of the anterior portion of the deltoids. The teres major synergizes this action. Externally rotate the shoulders by activating the infraspinatus and teres minor muscles of the rotator cuff. The posterior deltoids also assist in rotating the shoulders. Then engage the supinator muscles of the forearms to press the outer edges of the palms into the back. The biceps are also a supinator, so this action further aids to open the chest.

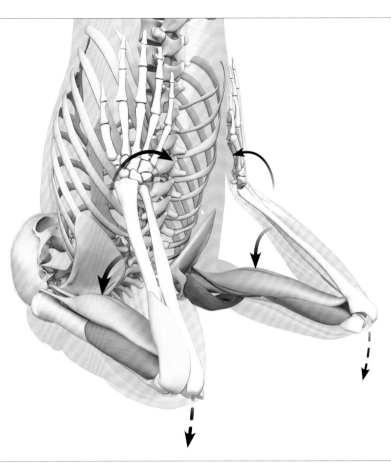

STEP 3 Balance the actions of the gluteus maximus, quadratus lumborum, and erector spinae by activating the hip flexors and abdominals. A cue for contracting the hip flexors is to bring the legs forward slightly. Then balance flexion and extension of the thighs so that the legs are held straight up in the air. This serves to stabilize the pelvis. Note how the abdominals connect the pelvis and the ribcage. Gently engage the rectus abdominis to balance the back extensors and stabilize the spine.

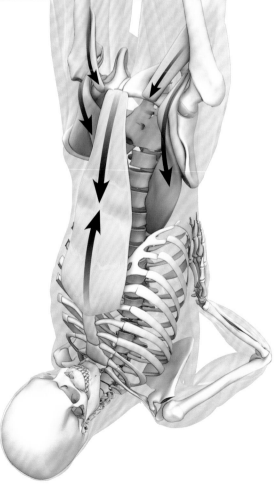

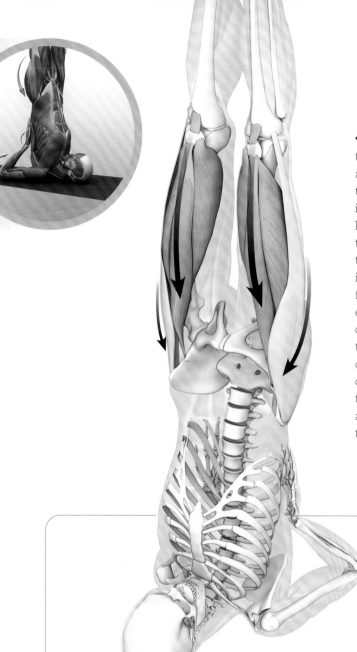

▲ STEP 4 Firmly contract the quadriceps to straighten the knees. Synergize this action and stabilize the knees by engaging the tensor fascia lata. This has the added effect of internally rotating the thighs and bringing the kneecaps back to a neutral position. Note that the kneecaps tend to rotate outward due to the action of the gluteus maximus described in Step 1. The cue for engaging the tensor fascia lata is to imagine pressing the outside edges of the feet against an immovable object. While the legs do not come apart, this stimulates contraction of the abductor component and accesses the secondary action of the tensor fascia lata, internally rotating the thighs. Another method of training this action is to place a belt snugly around the thighs and attempt to pull the legs apart.

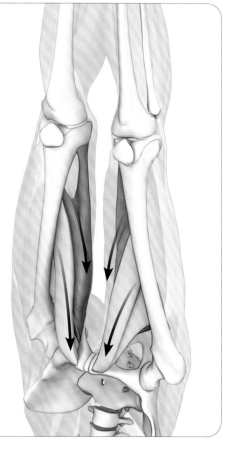

▶ STEP 5 Squeeze the knees together to engage the adductor group, stabilizing the legs in the air. The most posterior of this group is the adductor magnus. This muscle also synergizes the gluteus maximus in extending the femurs.

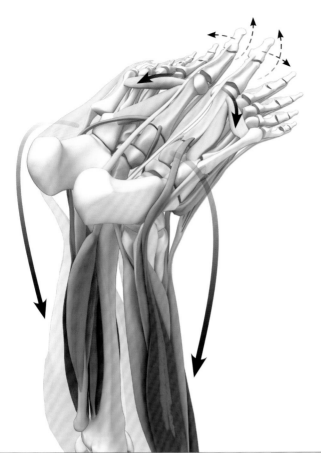

STEP 6 Evert the ankles by contracting the peroneus longus and brevis muscles. Then balance this action by slightly inverting the ankles using the tibialis posterior. This combination of opposing forces creates a bandha that stabilizes the feet.

Activate the tibialis anterior muscles to draw the tops of the feet toward the shins. Extend the toes. Then try flexing and adducting the big toes to deepen the foot arches. This engages the flexors hallucis longus and brevis and adductor hallucis. You can gain awareness of these muscles before going into the pose by pressing the fleshy part of the big toe into the floor and attempting to drag it toward the second toe. Feel how these combined actions dynamize the longitudinal arches of the feet. The tibialis posterior also contributes to this (in addition to inverting and stabilizing the ankles).

SUMMARY The pectoralis major and minor, the anterior deltoids, the coracobrachialis, and the subscapularis muscles all stretch. The biceps also stretch, although they are described as contracting in Step 2. This is an eccentric type of contraction. The upper portion of the erector spinae lengthens by flexing the neck.

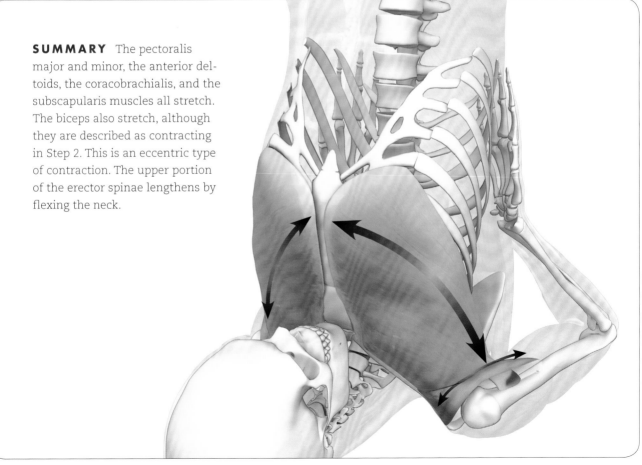

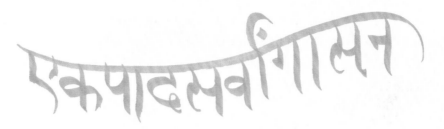

EKA PADA SARVANGASANA

ONE-LEGGED SHOULDER STAND

EKA PADA SARVANGASANA SHARES THE SAME BENEFITS AS THE OTHER inversions and adds a stretch of the gluteals, hamstrings, and gastrocnemius/soleus on the leg that is lowering to the floor. It also strengthens the posterior kinetic chain on the side of the leg that is raised. Leaning back into the hands opens the chest in the same manner as conventional Sarvangasana.

Nothing in the body moves independently. For example, lowering the leg can result in that side of the body squashing and the cervical spine hyperflexing. Anticipate these types of effects and plan to counteract them as you lower the leg. Lean into the hands to open the chest. Expand the side of the body that is prone to collapse by engaging the lower back muscles to arch and lift the lumbar. The psoas major of the flexing hip will synergize these muscles in supporting the lumbar region. Similarly, engage the oblique abdominals on the side of the leg that remains in the air. This will counterbalance the squash of the trunk on the other side.

BASIC JOINT POSITIONS

- The shoulders extend and externally rotate.
- The elbows flex.
- The forearms supinate.
- The trunk extends.
- The cervical spine flexes.
- The lifted-leg hip extends, adducts, and internally rotates.
- The lowered-leg hip flexes.
- The knees extend.
- The raised-leg ankle is neutral or plantar flexes slightly.
- The lowered-leg ankle dorsiflexes.
- The feet evert.
- The toes extend.

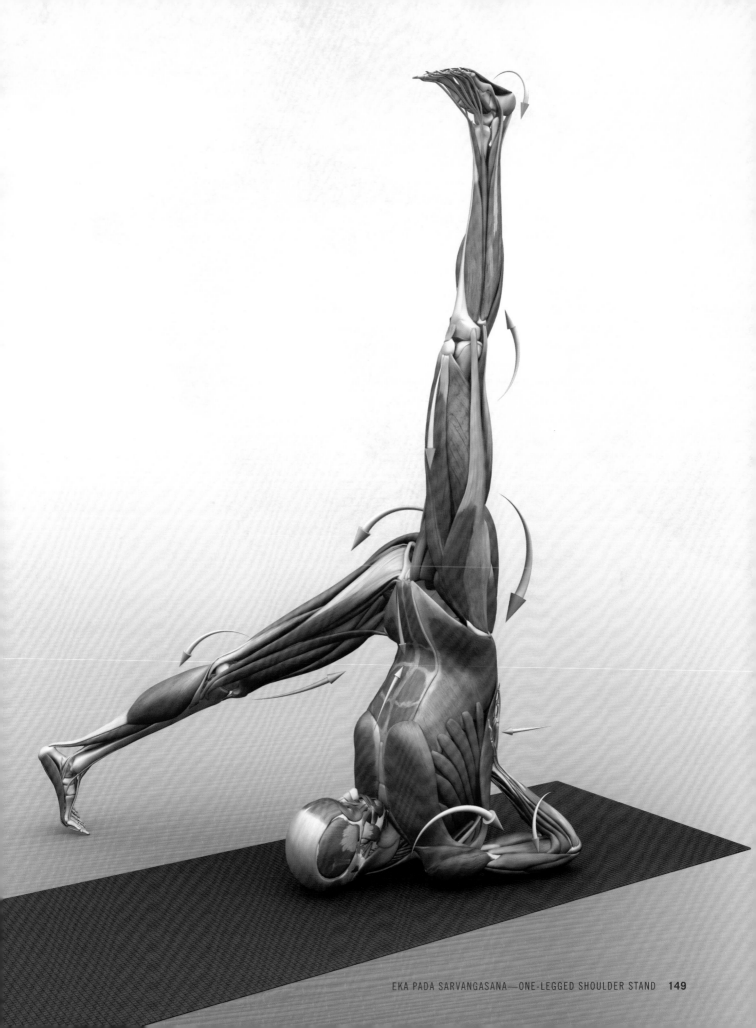

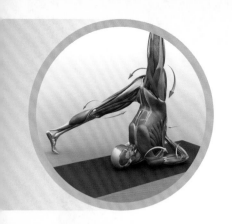

Eka Pada Sarvangasana Preparation

Prepare for the asana by stretching the hamstrings, gluteals, and hip flexors. Use poses such as Parsvottanasana and Hanumanasana to create length in these muscles. Stretch the pectorals and anterior deltoids to prepare the shoulders for drawing the elbows toward the floor in the final pose.

Then go into Sarvangasana. Lever the chest open by leaning back into the hands and pressing the backs of the elbows into the mat. Then lower one leg. Use a chair in the beginning. As you gain stability and flexibility, lower the leg further, using the psoas muscle to flex the hip. Raise the leg up again when you are ready to come out of the pose. Brace the back with the hands before coming down into Halasana; then use control to roll out of the pose and onto the back. Rest there for a few moments to allow the cardiovascular system to readjust.

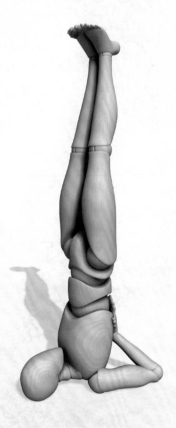

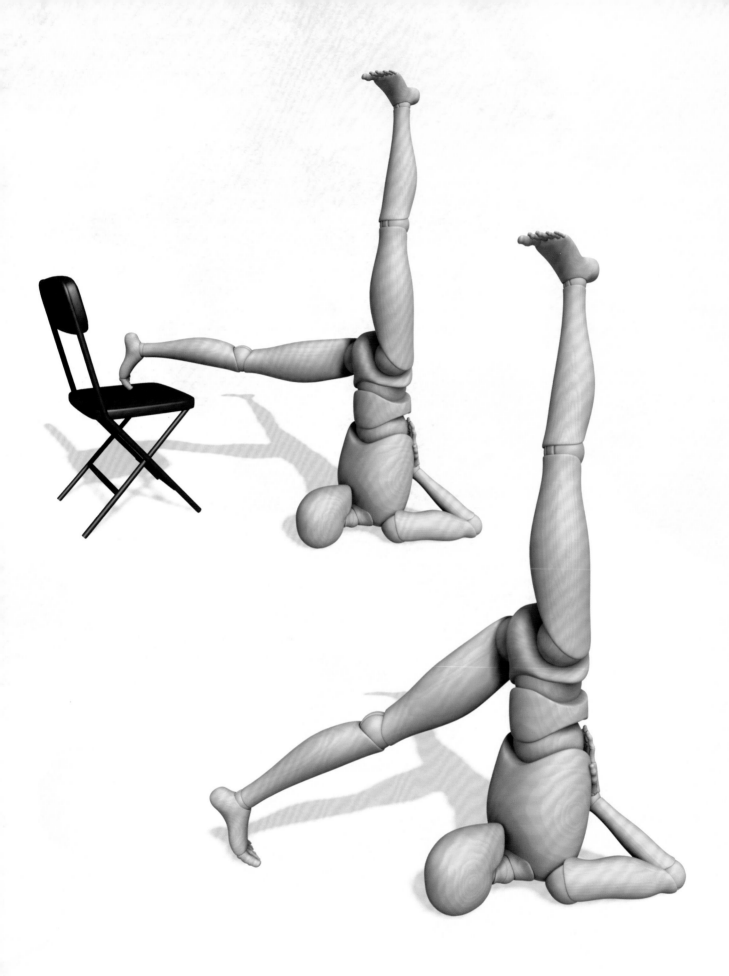

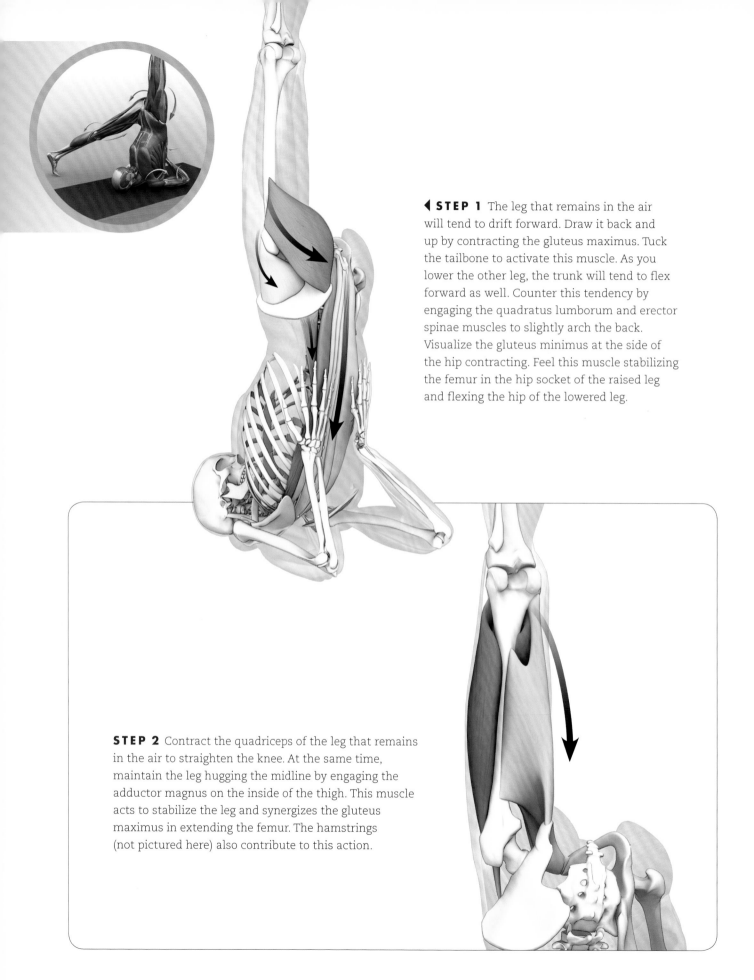

◀ **STEP 1** The leg that remains in the air will tend to drift forward. Draw it back and up by contracting the gluteus maximus. Tuck the tailbone to activate this muscle. As you lower the other leg, the trunk will tend to flex forward as well. Counter this tendency by engaging the quadratus lumborum and erector spinae muscles to slightly arch the back. Visualize the gluteus minimus at the side of the hip contracting. Feel this muscle stabilizing the femur in the hip socket of the raised leg and flexing the hip of the lowered leg.

STEP 2 Contract the quadriceps of the leg that remains in the air to straighten the knee. At the same time, maintain the leg hugging the midline by engaging the adductor magnus on the inside of the thigh. This muscle acts to stabilize the leg and synergizes the gluteus maximus in extending the femur. The hamstrings (not pictured here) also contribute to this action.

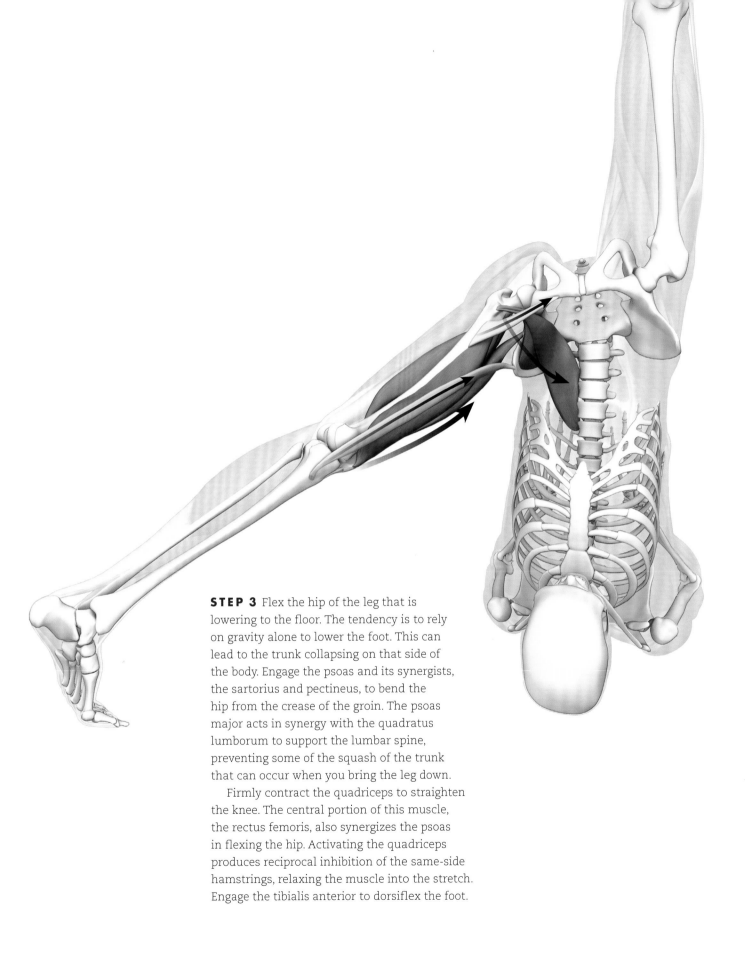

STEP 3 Flex the hip of the leg that is lowering to the floor. The tendency is to rely on gravity alone to lower the foot. This can lead to the trunk collapsing on that side of the body. Engage the psoas and its synergists, the sartorius and pectineus, to bend the hip from the crease of the groin. The psoas major acts in synergy with the quadratus lumborum to support the lumbar spine, preventing some of the squash of the trunk that can occur when you bring the leg down.

Firmly contract the quadriceps to straighten the knee. The central portion of this muscle, the rectus femoris, also synergizes the psoas in flexing the hip. Activating the quadriceps produces reciprocal inhibition of the same-side hamstrings, relaxing the muscle into the stretch. Engage the tibialis anterior to dorsiflex the foot.

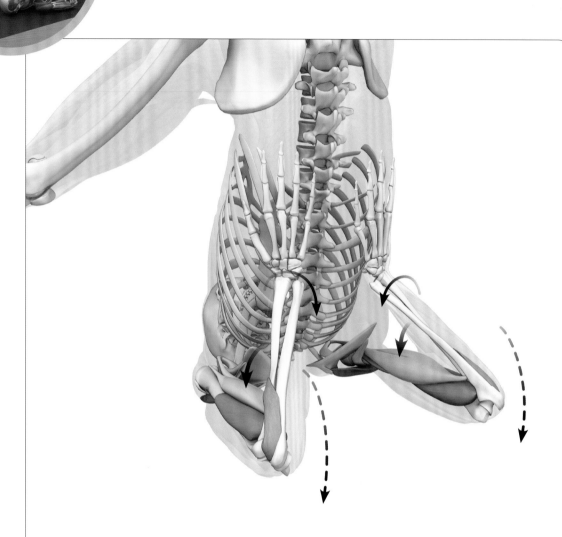

STEP 4 Activate the biceps and brachialis muscles to flex the elbows and press the palms into the back. Then lean back into the hands and feel how this opens the chest. Supinate the forearms to spread the weight from the index finger side across the palms. Press the backs of the elbows into the mat by firmly engaging the posterior deltoids. This extends the upper arm bones (the humeri) and aids to open the chest. Externally rotate the shoulders by contracting the infraspinatus and teres minor muscles (not pictured here). The posterior deltoids synergize this action.

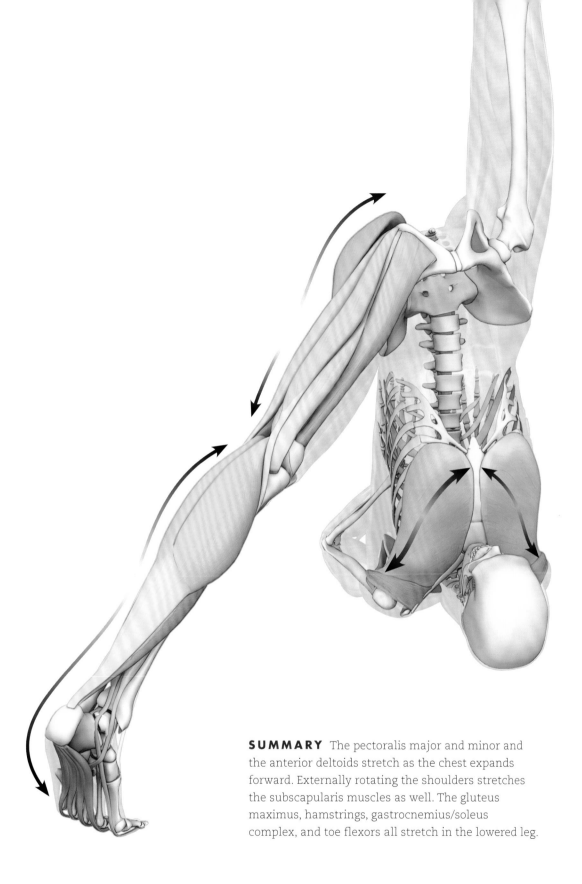

SUMMARY The pectoralis major and minor and the anterior deltoids stretch as the chest expands forward. Externally rotating the shoulders stretches the subscapularis muscles as well. The gluteus maximus, hamstrings, gastrocnemius/soleus complex, and toe flexors all stretch in the lowered leg.

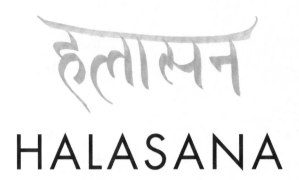

HALASANA

PLOUGH POSE

HALASANA IS A SHOULDER STAND VARIATION THAT COMBINES OPENING THE chest with stretching the posterior kinetic chain. It shares many of the same potential benefits as the other inverted postures, such as improved venous return and cardiac output and increased parasympathetic outflow.

Halasana is typically performed at the end of the practice, during the cool down phase leading to relaxation. The legs are taken over the head, flexing the hips. Such a position brings the center of gravity forward. Accordingly, care must be taken to maintain most of the body weight on the shoulders and arms and to avoid hyperflexion of the neck. Use a blanket to support the shoulders and allow the head to hang over the edge. This takes the neck out of hyperflexion and frees the cervical spine from excessive compression.

As in other inversions where the legs are brought to the floor (such as Eka Pada Sarvangasana), there is a tendency to collapse the torso and let gravity do the work of bending the hips. Avoid this by actively engaging the hip flexors, including the powerful psoas muscle. The psoas major also supports the lumbar spine. Synergize this action by contracting the quadratus lumborum and lower back muscles to create a slight arch in the lumbar. Lean into the hands and press them into the back to expand the chest; this draws the center of gravity away from the neck, aiding to protect the cervical spine.

BASIC JOINT POSITIONS

- The hips flex and adduct.
- The knees extend.
- The ankles dorsiflex.
- The feet evert.
- The toes extend.

- The trunk flexes.
- The shoulders extend and externally rotate.
- The elbows flex.
- The forearms supinate.

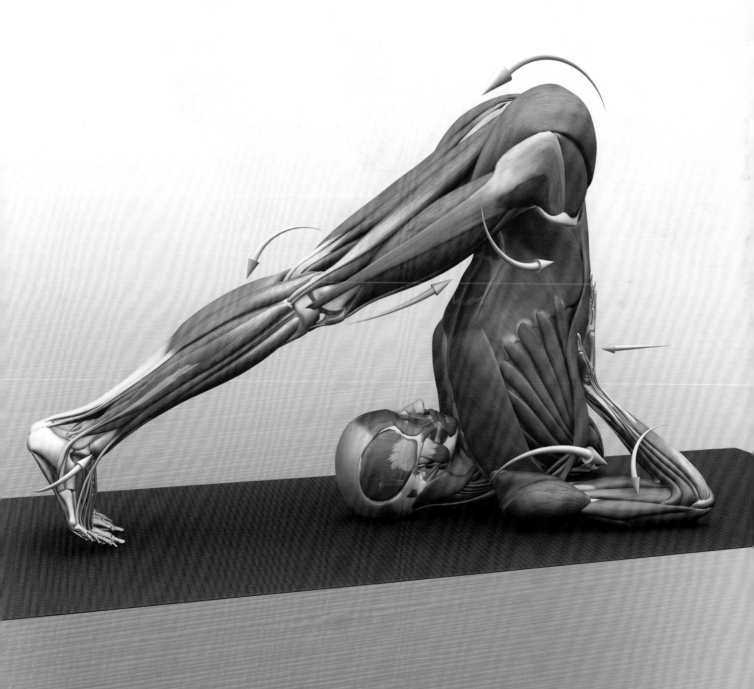

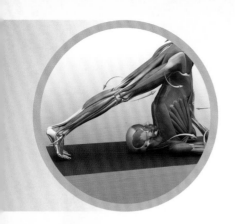

Halasana Preparation

Use poses such as Kurmasana and Paschimottanasana (below) to stretch the lower back muscles.

Roll over onto the shoulders, using a blanket for support as shown. Rest the tops of the thighs onto a chair or bring the feet onto the wall. Then progress to full Halasana by placing the feet on the floor. Carefully roll out of the pose by placing the hands palms down on the mat behind you; then draw the knees into the chest and bring the small of the back, then the pelvis, and finally the legs onto the floor. Place a blanket under the head and rest for several moments before coming out of the pose. This allows the cardiovascular system to readjust.

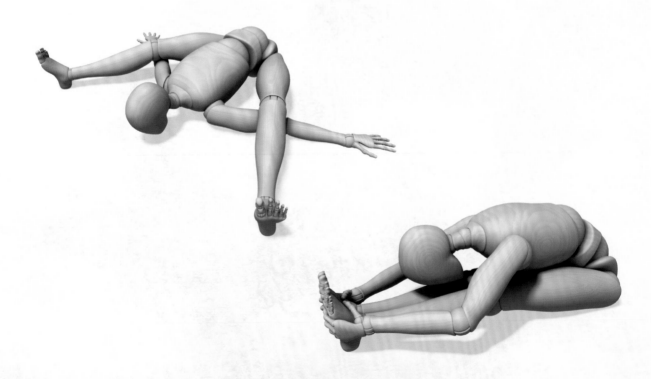

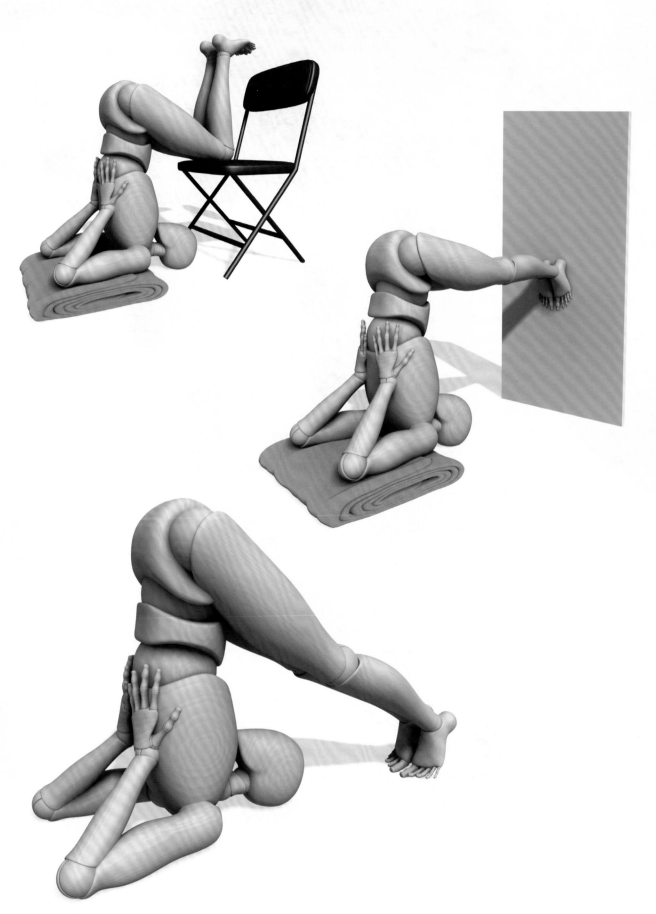

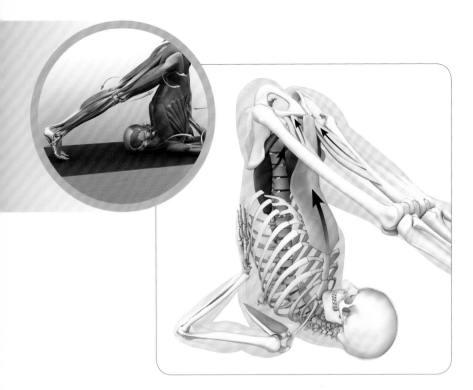

STEP 1 Draw the legs over the head to flex the trunk. Engage the psoas and its synergists, the pectineus and adductors longus and brevis, to flex the hips. Visualize the gluteus minimus at the sides of the hips contracting to synergize the hip flexors. The psoas is connected neurologically to the quadratus lumborum in the lumbar spine region. These two muscles work together to support and lift the small of the back. The adductors help to keep the legs together. Gently engage the rectus abdominis to flex the trunk. Note the attachment of this muscle on the front of the pelvis (the pubic symphysis). The pull of the rectus abdominis opposes the action of the psoas, creating a bandha that aids to stabilize the pelvis.

STEP 2 Arch the lower back by contracting the erector spinae and quadratus lumborum. Because these muscles are also stretching in the pose, this is an eccentric contraction. Leaning back into the hands prepares the chest for expansion in Step 3.

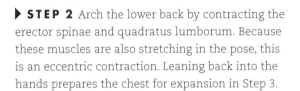

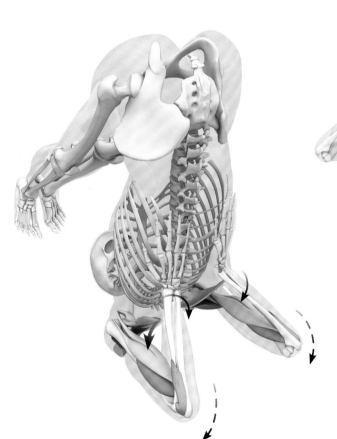

STEP 3 Flex the elbows and press the palms of the hands into the back by contracting the biceps and brachialis muscles. There is a tendency for the weight to shift onto the index finger sides of the hands. Balance this by supinating the forearms to spread the weight across the palms. Press the backs of the elbows into the mat by contracting the posterior deltoids. These muscles combine with the infraspinatus and teres minor muscles to externally rotate the shoulders, aiding to open the chest.

▶ **STEP 4** Contract the quadriceps to straighten the knees. The tensor fascia lata synergizes this action and contributes to flexing the hips (with the psoas). Note that the pull of the stretching gluteus maximus can externally rotate the thighs. Counter this by further engaging the tensor fascia lata. The cue for this is to attempt to drag the feet apart on the mat. The feet won't move, but the thighs will turn in and bring the kneecaps back to a neutral position. Bring the tops of the feet toward the shins to dorsiflex the ankles. This engages the tibialis anterior, producing reciprocal inhibition of the gastrocnemius and soleus muscles at the backs of the calves.

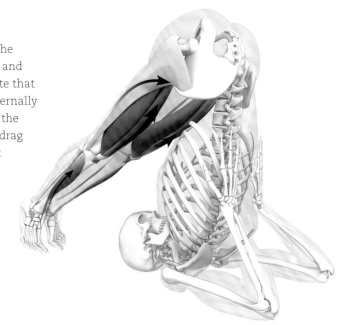

STEP 5 Evert the ankles by contracting the peroneus longus and brevis muscles. Balance this action by engaging the tibialis posterior, which acts to invert the ankles. These two opposing forces create a bandha that stabilizes the lower legs. Use the toe extensors to draw the toes toward the shins. All of the muscles illustrated in this step dynamize the arches of the feet and stimulate the minor chakras located in the soles.

▶ **SUMMARY** The chest opens, stretching the pectoralis major and minor and the anterior deltoids. Externally rotating the shoulders also stretches the subscapularis muscles of the rotator cuff. The entire back of the body lengthens, including the erector spinae, quadratus lumborum, gluteus maximus, hamstrings, and gastrocnemius/soleus complex. The toe flexors at the bottoms of the feet also stretch.

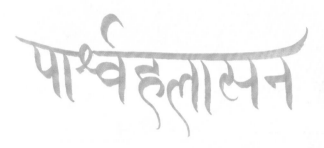

PARSVA HALASANA

REVOLVING PLOUGH POSE

PARSVA HALASANA COMBINES AN INVERSION, A TWIST, AND A STRETCH OF THE posterior kinetic chain. It shares the same potential benefits as other inversions, including beneficial effects on the autonomic nervous system. It has the additional effect of a kriya that is formed across the abdomen by the twist.

Care must be taken to bear the weight of the body on the shoulders and arms. Do not place the weight on the neck, as this can hyperflex the cervical spine and cause injury. Note that the shoulder you are twisting away from will tend to come forward while the other shoulder tends to roll back in the direction of the twist. Counter this by pressing the elbow firmly into the mat on the side you are twisting away from. The muscles section below provides cues for how to do this. Remember that you can enhance the effect of twisting postures by turning the shoulder and hip girdles in opposite directions.

Avoid collapsing the torso on the side that the legs turn toward. Engage the opposite-side abdominals and lower back muscles to prevent this. In addition, use the psoas major and quadratus lumborum to arch the lower back, creating length in the trunk.

BASIC JOINT POSITIONS

- The hips flex and adduct.
- The knees extend.
- The ankles dorsiflex.
- The feet evert.
- The toes extend.

- The trunk flexes and rotates.
- The shoulders extend and externally rotate.
- The elbows flex.
- The forearms supinate.

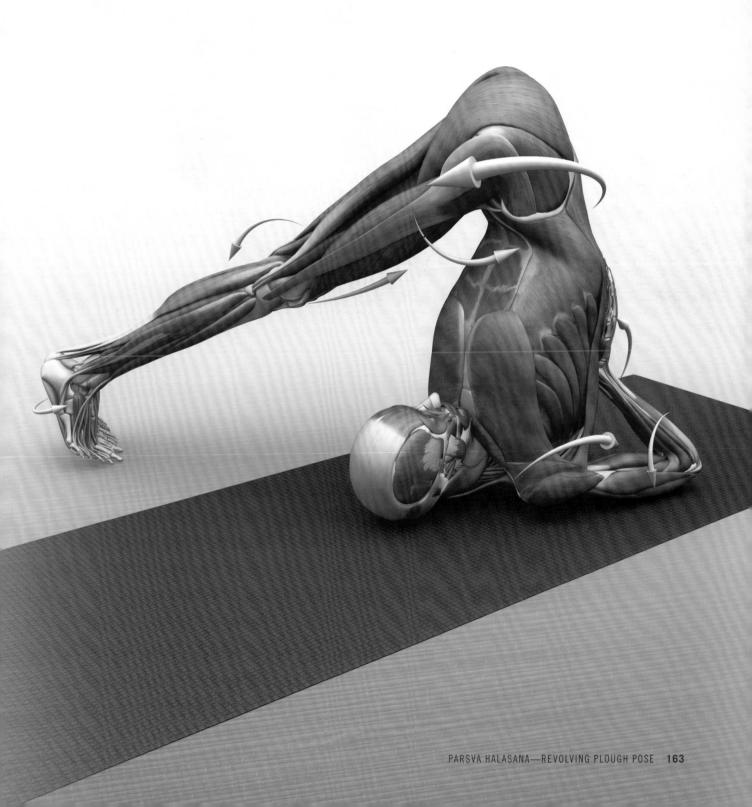

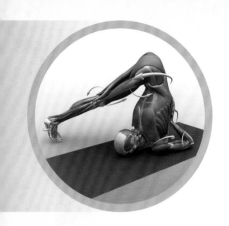

Parsva Halasana Preparation

Practice a pose such as Kurmasana or Upavistha Konasana to lengthen the lower back muscles and prepare the posterior kinetic chain for the stretch of Parsva Halasana. Additionally, use a twist such as Marichyasana III to prepare the spinal rotators.

Begin with Halasana. Lean into the hands, and press the palms into the back to open the chest. This aids to take the weight away from the cervical spine. Carefully walk the feet over to one side to rotate the lower body away from the upper. Resist with the shoulder on the side you are twisting away from by pressing the elbow into the mat. When the feet reach their final position in the twist, they will be uneven. Bend the knee slightly (of the foot that is further away) to walk that foot in line with the other one. Then, with this same foot fixed on the floor, contract the quadriceps to straighten the knee. Note how this balances the pelvis.

Re-establish Halasana before going to the other side. Return to center and then roll out of the pose. Rest on your back for a few moments to allow the cardiovascular system to readjust.

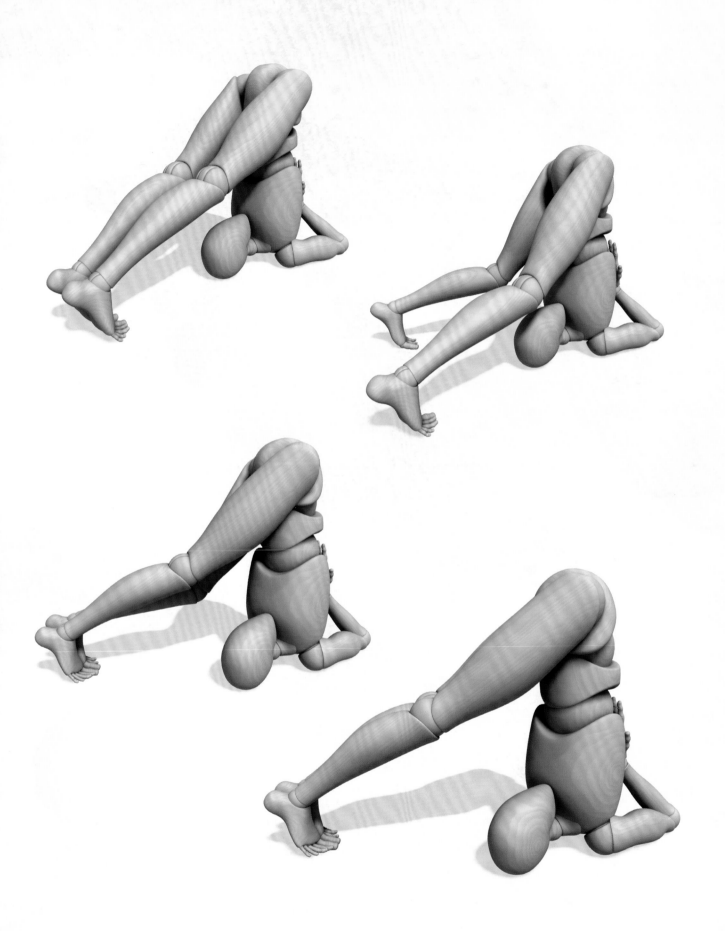

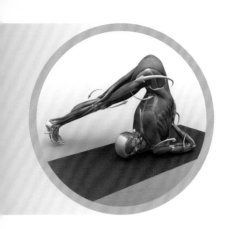

▶ **STEP 1** Flex the hips by contracting the psoas, pectineus, and adductors longus and brevis. Visualize the gluteus minimus contracting on the sides of the pelvis to aid in this action. Engage the rectus abdominis and oblique abdominals to squeeze and turn the torso. Note that the psoas major will also synergize the quadratus lumborum in arching the lower back.

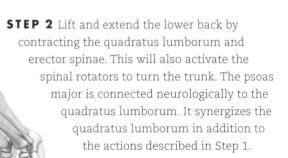

STEP 2 Lift and extend the lower back by contracting the quadratus lumborum and erector spinae. This will also activate the spinal rotators to turn the trunk. The psoas major is connected neurologically to the quadratus lumborum. It synergizes the quadratus lumborum in addition to the actions described in Step 1.

▶ **STEP 3** Press the palms of the hands into the back by bending the elbows. This contracts the biceps and brachialis muscles. Supinate the forearms to distribute the weight of the body evenly across the hands. The biceps aid in this action. Engage the posterior deltoids and teres major muscles to press the elbows into the mat. The posterior deltoids also synergize the infraspinatus and teres minor muscles to externally rotate the shoulders. Note that the shoulder on the side the legs are turning away from will drift forward. Counter this by activating all of the muscles described above more forcefully on that side.

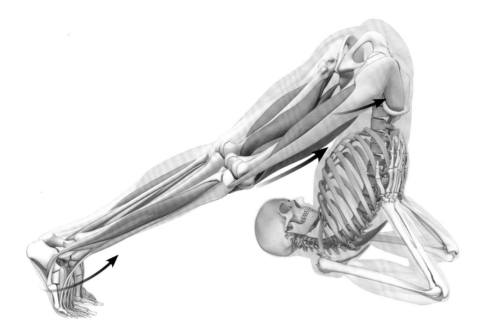

STEP 4 Straighten the knees by engaging the quadriceps. The tensor fascia lata will synergize extending the knees and also aid in flexing the hips. A cue for contracting this muscle is to attempt to drag the feet apart on the mat (gently). You will feel an additional benefit of internally rotating the thighs, which brings the kneecaps to a neutral position.

Activate the peroneus longus and brevis muscles at the sides of the lower legs to evert the feet. Balance this action by engaging the tibialis posterior to produce an inversion force. These opposing actions create a gentle bandha at the ankles. Contract the tibialis anterior muscles to dorsiflex the feet. This draws the tops of the feet toward the shins, also creating reciprocal inhibition of the gastrocnemius and soleus muscles on the calves. Extend the toes. All of these actions work together to stabilize the feet and open the soles, stimulating the minor chakras located in this region.

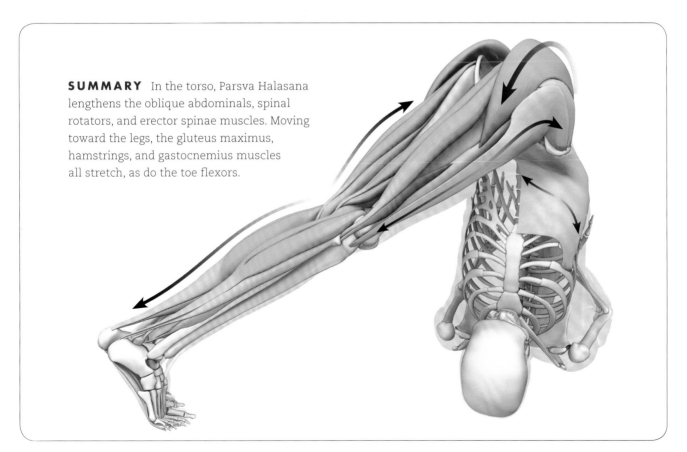

SUMMARY In the torso, Parsva Halasana lengthens the oblique abdominals, spinal rotators, and erector spinae muscles. Moving toward the legs, the gluteus maximus, hamstrings, and gastocnemius muscles all stretch, as do the toe flexors.

RESTORATIVE POSES
BALASANA CHILD'S POSE

Inversions can cause increased parasympathetic outflow from the central nervous system, resulting in lowered heart rate and blood pressure. Accordingly, it is necessary to allow the cardiovascular system to re-equilibrate following inverted postures. Use intermediary poses such as Balasana (Child's Pose) to avoid light-headedness before coming up from the mat.

Flex the hips and abduct them so that the knees come to the outside of the trunk. Bend forward and flex the shoulders to place the hands on the floor. Rest the head on the mat. You can also add the variation shown, in which a weight is placed on the back to aid in relaxing the erector spinae and quadratus lumborum muscles.

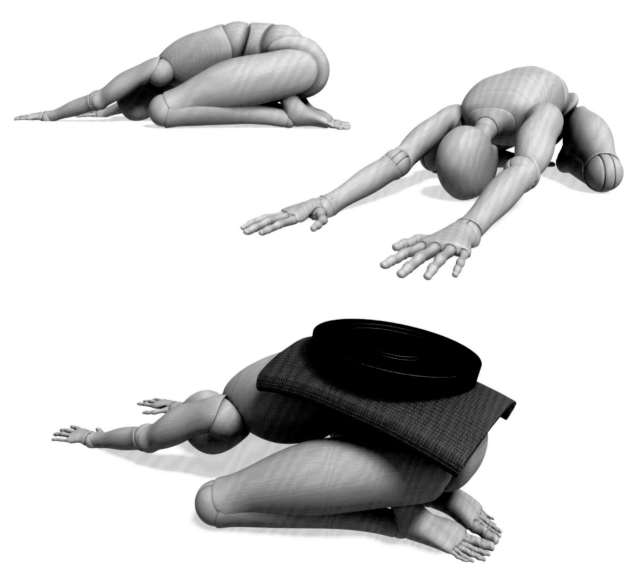

VIPARITA KARANI & SAVASANA
LEGS-UP-THE-WALL POSE & CORPSE POSE

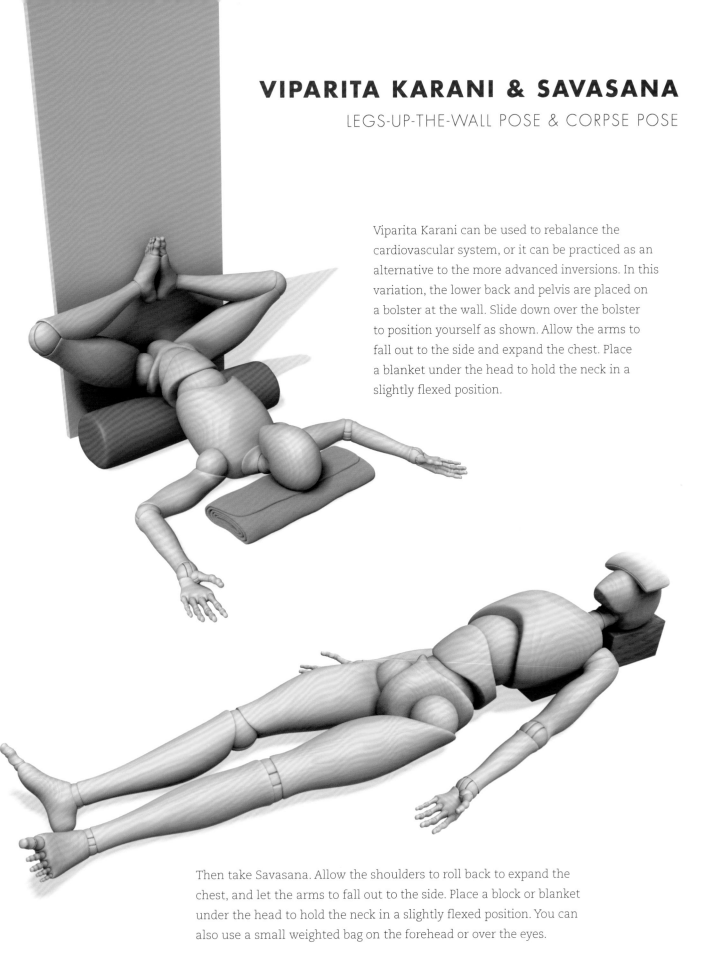

Viparita Karani can be used to rebalance the cardiovascular system, or it can be practiced as an alternative to the more advanced inversions. In this variation, the lower back and pelvis are placed on a bolster at the wall. Slide down over the bolster to position yourself as shown. Allow the arms to fall out to the side and expand the chest. Place a blanket under the head to hold the neck in a slightly flexed position.

Then take Savasana. Allow the shoulders to roll back to expand the chest, and let the arms to fall out to the side. Place a block or blanket under the head to hold the neck in a slightly flexed position. You can also use a small weighted bag on the forehead or over the eyes.

MOVEMENT
INDEX

MOVEMENT INDEX

Movements of the body have specific names. It is important to learn these names, both for teaching others yoga and for analyzing the muscles that produce the positions of the body. As a yoga teacher, it is always better to communicate your instructions in terminology that students can easily understand. Know the scientific names of the movements and have clear explanations to describe the movements in layperson's terms. Make your instructions as precise and uncomplicated as you can.

Remember that muscles contract to position the joints and appendages in the pose. If you know the joint positions, you can analyze which muscles to engage to produce the asana. With this knowledge comes the ability to use precise cues to communicate how to sculpt and stabilize the body in the pose, stretch the correct muscles, and create bandhas. Thus, unlocking the asana begins with a clear understanding of body movements.

There are six basic movements of the body: Flexion, Extension, Adduction, Abduction, Internal Rotation, and External Rotation. These movements take place in three planes, as shown here. The anatomic position is the reference point to define the direction of movement.

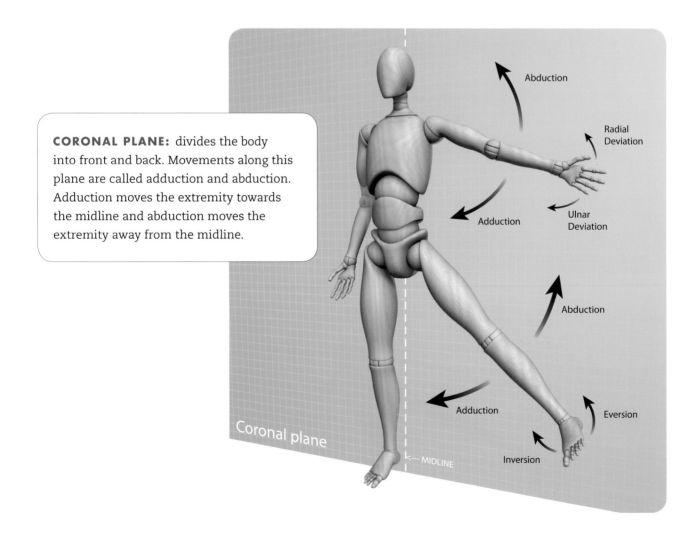

CORONAL PLANE: divides the body into front and back. Movements along this plane are called adduction and abduction. Adduction moves the extremity towards the midline and abduction moves the extremity away from the midline.

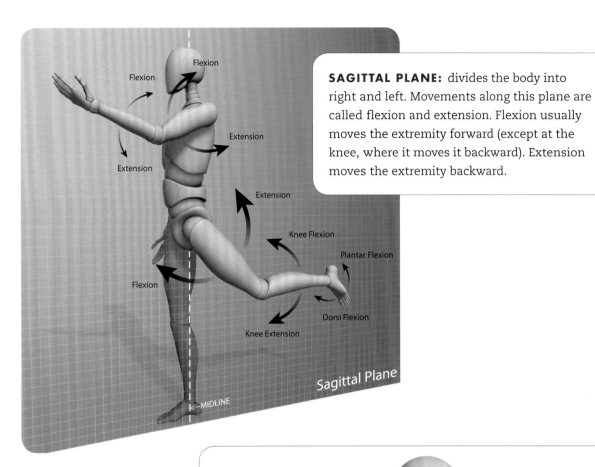

SAGITTAL PLANE: divides the body into right and left. Movements along this plane are called flexion and extension. Flexion usually moves the extremity forward (except at the knee, where it moves it backward). Extension moves the extremity backward.

TRANSVERSE PLANE: divides the body into upper and lower halves. Movement along this plane is called rotation. Rotation is further classified as internal (towards the midline) and external (away from the midline). Internal and external rotation are also referred to as medial and lateral rotation, respectively.

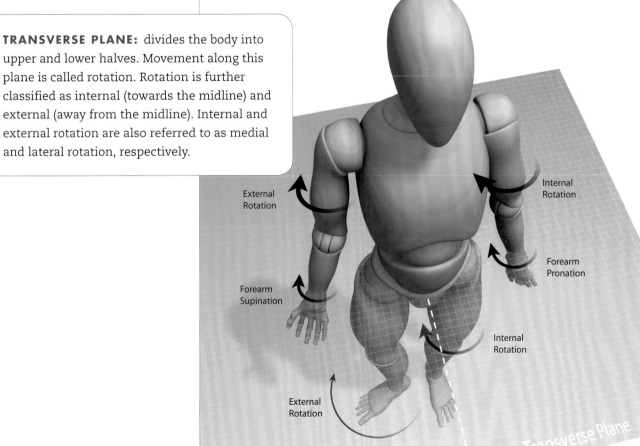

MOVEMENT INDEX

Eka Pada Bakasana I and Eka Pada Sarvangasana are presented as examples of how to analyze the basic joint positions in a yoga pose. The order represents the sequence of movements that create the form of the pose.

1 The shoulders flex, adduct, and externally rotate.

2 The elbows partly extend.

3 The forearms pronate.

4 The hip flexes and adducts.

5 The knee flexes.

6 The foot everts.

7 The trunk flexes.

8 The hip extends.

9 The knee extends.

10 The ankle plantar flexes.

11 The neck extends.

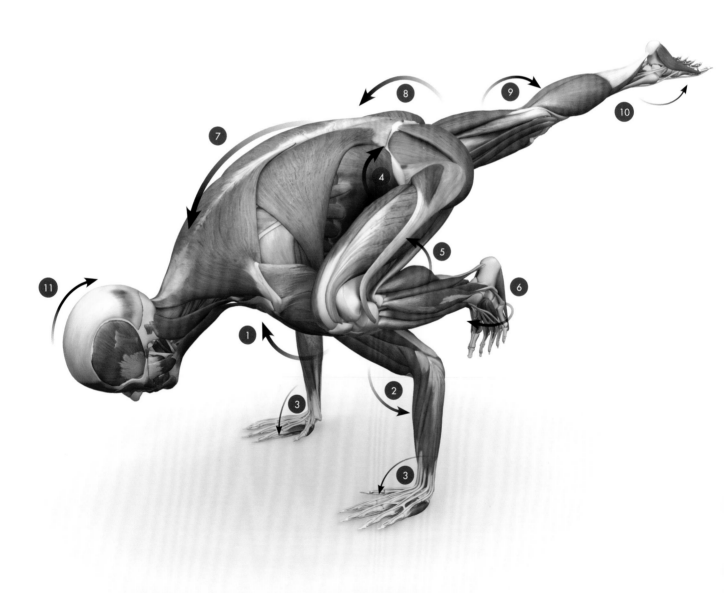

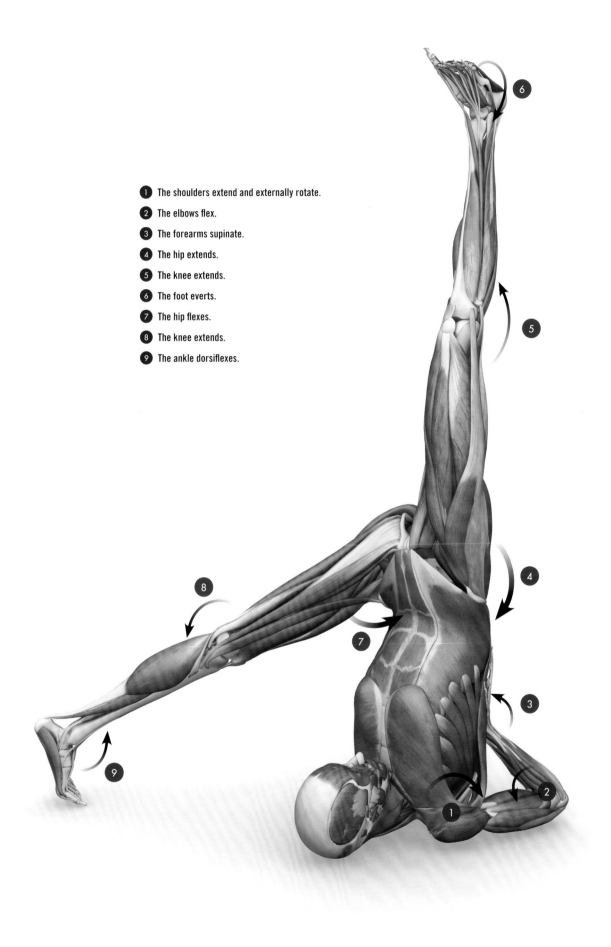

1 The shoulders extend and externally rotate.

2 The elbows flex.

3 The forearms supinate.

4 The hip extends.

5 The knee extends.

6 The foot everts.

7 The hip flexes.

8 The knee extends.

9 The ankle dorsiflexes.

MOVEMENT TABLES

Neck

Muscle	Flexion	Extension	Lateral Flexion	Lateral Extension	Rotation
Semispinalis capitis		●	●	●	●
Splenius capitis		●	●	●	●
Sternocleidomastoid	●		●	●	●
Levator scapulae		●	●	●	
Trapezius		●	●	●	●

Trunk

Muscle	Flexion	Extension	Lateral Flexion	Rotation
External oblique	●		●	●
Internal oblique	●		●	●
Rectus abdominis	●			
Spinalis thoracis		●		
Lateral intertransversi			●	
Interspinales		●		
Longissimus thoracis		●		
Iliocostalis lumborum		●		
Multifidus		●		
Rotatores		●		●
Quadratus lumborum		●	●	
Psoas major	●		●	
Iliacus	●		●	

Hip

Muscle	Flexion	Extension	Adduction	Abduction	Internal Rotation	External Rotation
Gluteus maximus		●				●
Gluteus medius	●	●		●	●	●
Gluteus minimus	●	●		●	●	●
Tensor fascia lata	●			●	●	
Psoas major	●					●
Iliacus	●					●
Rectus femoris	●			●		
Sartorius	●			●		●
Pectineus	●		●			●
Adductor magnus		●	●			●
Adductor longus	●		●			●
Adductor brevis	●		●			●
Gracilis	●		●			●
Piriformis				●		●
Gemellus superior				●		●
Gemellus inferior				●		●
Obturator internus				●		●
Obturator externus						●
Quadratus femoris			●			●
Semitendinosus		●			●	
Semimembranosus		●			●	
Biceps femoris		●				●

MOVEMENT TABLES

Knee

Muscle	Flexion	Extension	Internal Rotation	External Rotation
Vastus medialis		●		
Vastus lateralis		●		
Vastus intermedius		●		
Rectus femoris		●		
Sartorius	●			●
Semitendinosus	●		●	
Semimembranosus	●		●	
Biceps femoris	●			●
Gracilis	●		●	
Popliteus	●			
Gastrocnemius	●			

Lower Leg

Muscle	Ankle Plantar Flexion	Ankle Dorsiflexion	Foot Eversion	Foot Inversion	Toe Flexion	Toe Extension
Gastrocnemius	●					
Soleus	●					
Tibialis anterior		●		●		
Tibialis posterior	●			●		
Peroneus longus	●		●			
Peroneus brevis	●		●			
Peroneus tertius	●		●			
Flexor digitorum longus	●			●	●	
Flexor hallucis longus	●			●	●	
Extensor digitorum longus		●	●			●
Extensor hallucis longus		●		●		●

Foot

Muscle	Toe Flexion	Toe Extension	Toe Adduction	Toe Abduction
Flexor digitorum brevis	●			
Flexor hallucis brevis	●			
Flexor digiti minimi brevis	●			
Extensor digitorum brevis		●		
Extensor hallucis brevis		●		
Abductor digiti minimi				●
Abductor hallucis				●
Adductor hallucis			●	
Lumbricales	●	●	●	
Plantar interosseus	●		●	
Dorsal interosseus	●			●

Hand

Muscle	Flexion	Extension	Adduction	Abduction
Flexor digitorum superficialis	●			
Flexor digitorum profundus	●			
Flexor pollicis longus	●			
Flexor pollicis brevis	●			
Flexor digiti minimi brevis	●			
Extensor digitorum		●		
Extensor pollicis longus		●		
Extensor pollicis brevis		●		
Extensor indicis		●		
Extensor digiti minimi		●		
Abductor pollicis longus				●
Abductor pollicis brevis				●
Adductor pollicis			●	
Abductor digiti minimi				●
Lumbricales	●	●		
Dorsal interosseus	●	●	●	

MOVEMENT TABLES

Arm and Wrist

Muscle	Elbow Flexion	Elbow Extension	Forearm Pronation	Forearm Supination	Wrist Flexion	Wrist Extension	Wrist Ulnar Deviation	Wrist Radial Deviation
Biceps brachii	●			●				
Brachialis	●							
Triceps brachii		●						
Anconeus		●						
Brachioradialis	●							
Supinator				●				
Pronator teres			●					
Pronator quadratus			●					
Extensor carpi radialis longus						●		●
Extensor carpi radialis brevis						●		●
Extensor carpi ulnaris						●	●	
Flexor carpi radialis					●			●
Flexor carpi ulnaris					●		●	
Extensor digitorum						●		
Extensor pollicis brevis								●
Extensor pollicis longus				●				●
Abductor pollicis longus								●

Shoulder

Muscle	Retraction	Protraction	Elevation	Depression	Flexion	Extension	Adduction	Abduction	Internal Rotation	External Rotation
Rhomboids	●									
Serratus anterior		●	●					●		
Trapezius	●		●	●			●	●		
Levator scapulae		●	●							
Latissimus dorsi	●			●		●	●		●	
Teres major						●	●		●	
Pectoralis major				●	●		●		●	
Pectoralis minor		●		●						
Anterior deltoid					●				●	
Lateral deltoid								●		
Posterior deltoid						●				●
Supraspinatus								●		
Infraspinatus										●
Teres minor							●			●
Subscapularis									●	
Biceps brachii					●					
Coracobrachialis					●		●			
Triceps brachii						●	●			

ANATOMY
INDEX

ANATOMY INDEX
BONES

1. skull
2. mandible
3. cervical spine
4. thoracic spine
5. lumbar spine
6. sacrum
7. ilium bone (pelvis)
8. ischial tuberosity (sit bone)
9. femur
10. patella
11. tibia
12. fibula
13. ribs
14. sternum
15. clavicle
16. scapula
17. humerus
18. radius
19. ulna
20. hindfoot
21. midfoot
22. forefoot
23. carpals (wrist)
24. metacarpals
25. phalanges

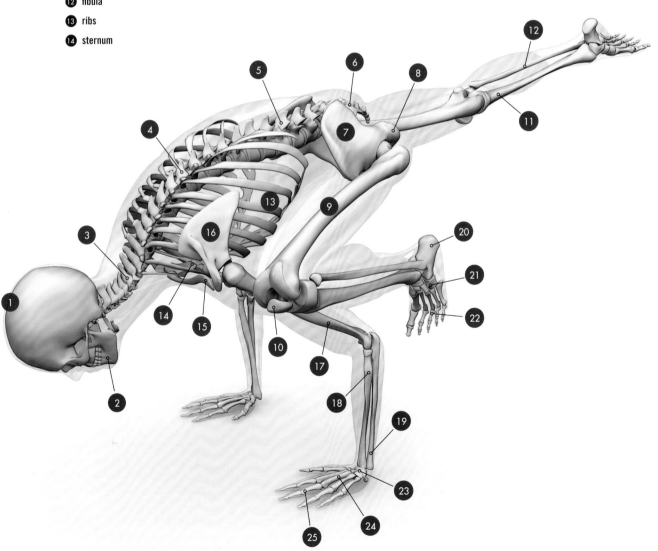

AXIAL AND APPENDICULAR SKELETONS

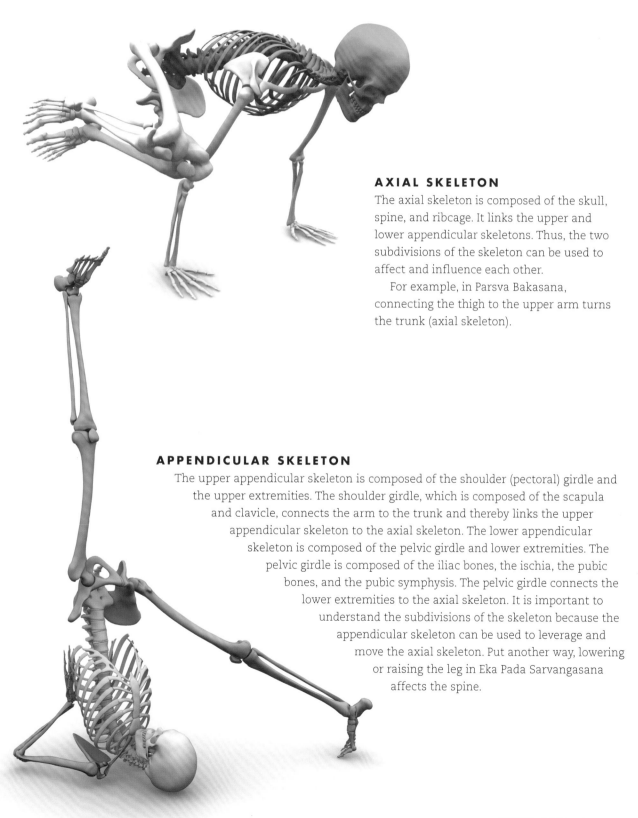

AXIAL SKELETON

The axial skeleton is composed of the skull, spine, and ribcage. It links the upper and lower appendicular skeletons. Thus, the two subdivisions of the skeleton can be used to affect and influence each other.

For example, in Parsva Bakasana, connecting the thigh to the upper arm turns the trunk (axial skeleton).

APPENDICULAR SKELETON

The upper appendicular skeleton is composed of the shoulder (pectoral) girdle and the upper extremities. The shoulder girdle, which is composed of the scapula and clavicle, connects the arm to the trunk and thereby links the upper appendicular skeleton to the axial skeleton. The lower appendicular skeleton is composed of the pelvic girdle and lower extremities. The pelvic girdle is composed of the iliac bones, the ischia, the pubic bones, and the pubic symphysis. The pelvic girdle connects the lower extremities to the axial skeleton. It is important to understand the subdivisions of the skeleton because the appendicular skeleton can be used to leverage and move the axial skeleton. Put another way, lowering or raising the leg in Eka Pada Sarvangasana affects the spine.

ANATOMY INDEX
MUSCLES

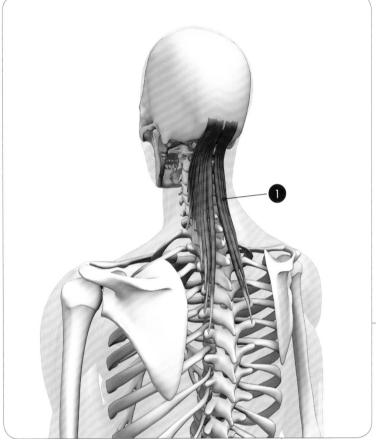

Legend

O = Origin. The proximal site where a muscle attaches to a bone.

I = Insertion. The distal site where a muscle attaches to a bone.

A = Action. The joint movement produced when the muscle contracts.

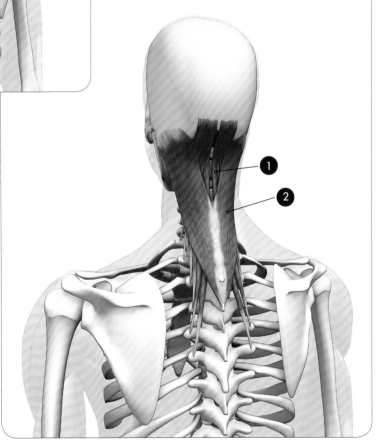

① Semispinalis capitis
- O: Transverse processes of lower cervical and upper thoracic vertebrae.
- I: Occipital bone.
- A: Extends head (tilts it back), assists in turning head.

② Splenius capitis
- O: Spinous processes of C7 and T1-4.
- I: Mastoid process of skull, behind ear.
- A: Extends head and neck; when one side contracts, laterally flexes neck; turns head toward side of individual muscle.

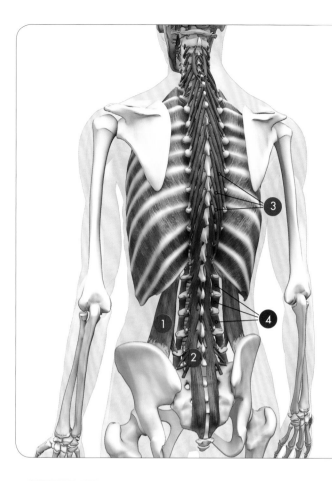

1 Quadratus lumborum
O: Posterior (back) of iliac crest.
I: Back part of rib 12, transverse processes of L1-4.
A: Laterally flexes spine (bends to side); extends and stabilizes lumbar spine; stabilizes rib 12, drawing it down during deep inhalation.

2 Multifidus
O: Back of sacrum and posterior superior iliac spine, transverse processes of lumbar, thoracic, and cervical vertebrae (all the way up the spine).
I: Two vertebrae above the vertebrae of origin; fibers are directed diagonally toward the midline and onto the spinous processes of the vertebrae of insertion.
A: Stabilizes spine during extension, flexion, and rotation.

3 Semispinalis thoracis
O: Transverse processes of T6-10.
I: Spinous processes of lower cervical and upper thoracic vertebrae.
A: Extends and rotates upper thoracic and lower cervical spine.

4 Lateral intertransversi
O: Transverse processes of lumbar vertebrae.
I: Transverse process of vertebrae immediately above vertebrae of origin.
A: Laterally flexes lumbar spine.

1 Serratus posterior superior
O: Ligamentum nuchae and spinous processes of C7-T4.
I: Ribs 2-5 on upper border.
A: Expands back of chest during deep inhalation by lifting ribs (is an accessory muscle of breathing).

2 Serratus posterior inferior
O: Spinous processes of T11-12, L1-3, thoracolumbar fascia.
I: Lower borders of ribs 9-12.
A: Stabilizes lower ribs during inhalation.

3 Spinalis thoracis
O: Transverse processes of T6-10.
I: Spinous processes of C6-7, T1-4.
A: Extends upper thoracic and lower cervical spine.

4 Longissimus thoracis
O: Posterior sacrum, spinous processes of T11-12, L1-5.
I: Transverse processes of T1-12, medial part of ribs 4-12.
A: Laterally flexes and extends spine, aids to expand chest during inhalation.

5 Iliocostalis lumborum
O: Posterior sacrum.
I: Posterior part of ribs 7-12.
A: Laterally flexes and extends lumbar spine.

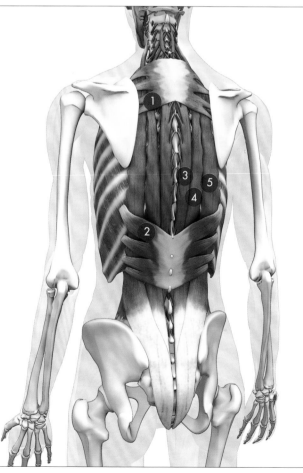

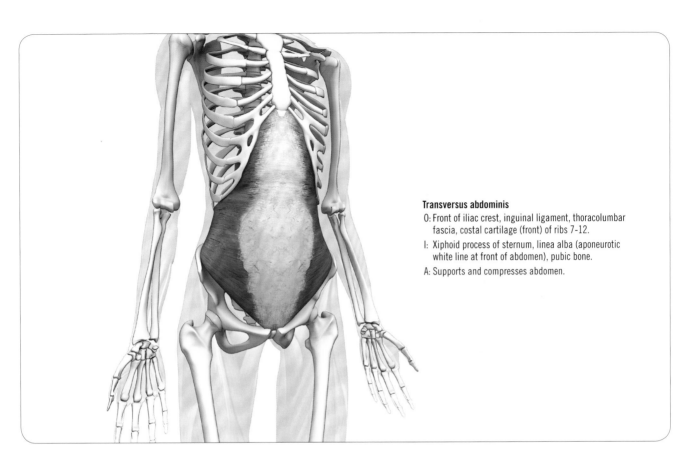

Transversus abdominis

O: Front of iliac crest, inguinal ligament, thoracolumbar fascia, costal cartilage (front) of ribs 7-12.

I: Xiphoid process of sternum, linea alba (aponeurotic white line at front of abdomen), pubic bone.

A: Supports and compresses abdomen.

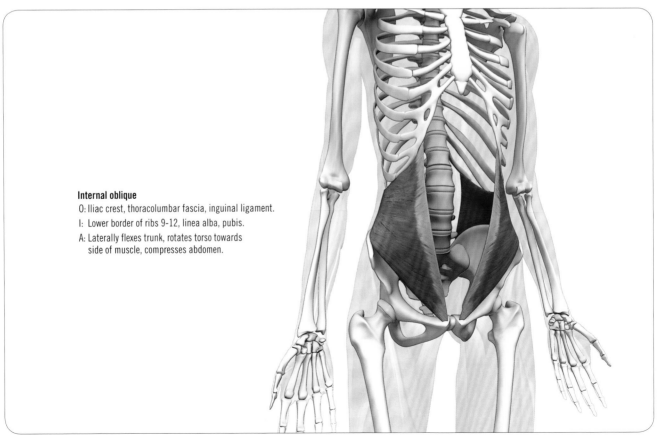

Internal oblique

O: Iliac crest, thoracolumbar fascia, inguinal ligament.

I: Lower border of ribs 9-12, linea alba, pubis.

A: Laterally flexes trunk, rotates torso towards side of muscle, compresses abdomen.

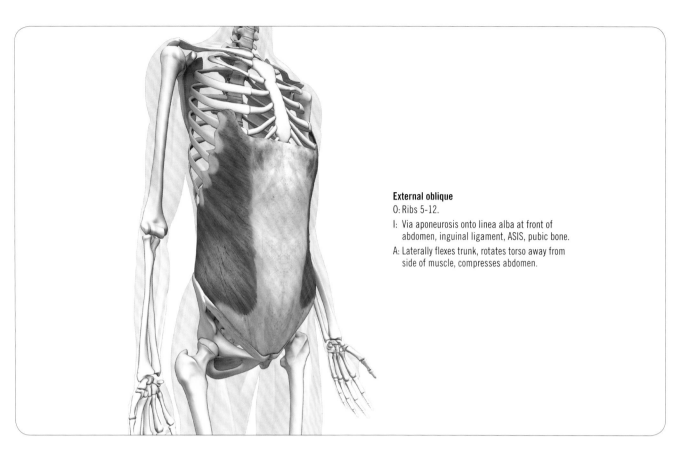

External oblique

O: Ribs 5-12.

I: Via aponeurosis onto linea alba at front of abdomen, inguinal ligament, ASIS, pubic bone.

A: Laterally flexes trunk, rotates torso away from side of muscle, compresses abdomen.

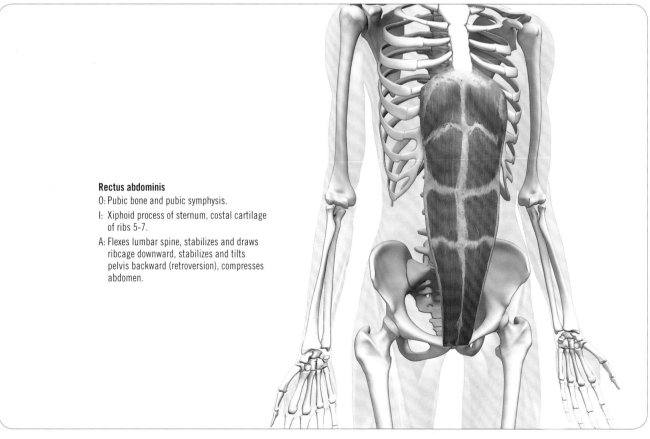

Rectus abdominis

O: Pubic bone and pubic symphysis.

I: Xiphoid process of sternum, costal cartilage of ribs 5-7.

A: Flexes lumbar spine, stabilizes and draws ribcage downward, stabilizes and tilts pelvis backward (retroversion), compresses abdomen.

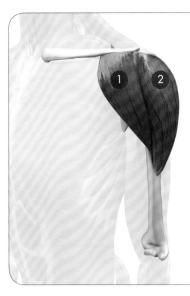

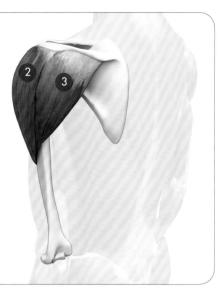

1 **Anterior deltoid**

O: Front and top of lateral third of clavicle.

I: Deltoid tuberosity on outer surface of humeral shaft.

A: Forward flexes and internally rotates humerus.

2 **Lateral deltoid**

O: Lateral border of acromion process of scapula.

I: Deltoid tuberosity on outer surface of humeral shaft.

A: Abducts humerus following initiation of movement by supraspinatus muscle of rotator cuff.

3 **Posterior deltoid**

O: Spine of scapula.

I: Deltoid tuberosity on outer surface of humeral shaft.

A: Extends and externally rotates humerus.

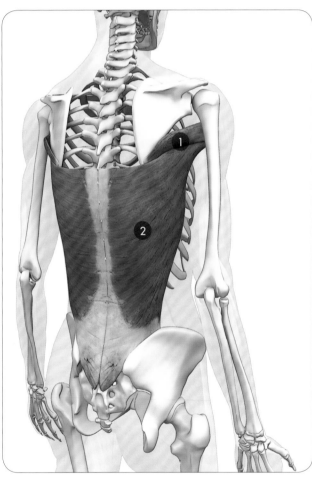

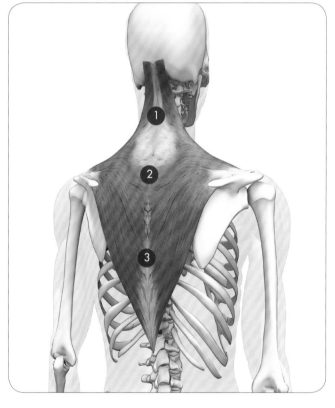

1 **Teres major**

O: Lower lateral border of scapula.

I: Bicipital groove of humerus.

A: Adducts and internally rotates humerus.

2 **Latissimus dorsi**

O: Thoracolumbar fascia, posterior portion of iliac crest, ribs 9-12, inferior border of scapula.

I: Bicipital groove of humerus.

A: Extends, adducts, and internally rotates humerus.

1 **Upper trapezius**

O: Occipital bone, ligamentum nuchae.

I: Upper border of spine of scapula.

A: Elevates (lifts) shoulder girdle, with lower trapezius rotates scapula to lift arm overhead.

2 **Middle trapezius**

O: Spinous processes of C7-T7.

I: Medial edge of acromion, posterior part of lateral third of clavicle.

A: Adducts (retracts) scapula.

3 **Lower trapezius**

O: Spinous processes of T8-12.

I: Medial edge of acromion, posterior part of lateral third of clavicle.

A: Depresses scapula, aids to hold body in arm balancing, with upper trapezius rotates scapula to lift arm overhead.

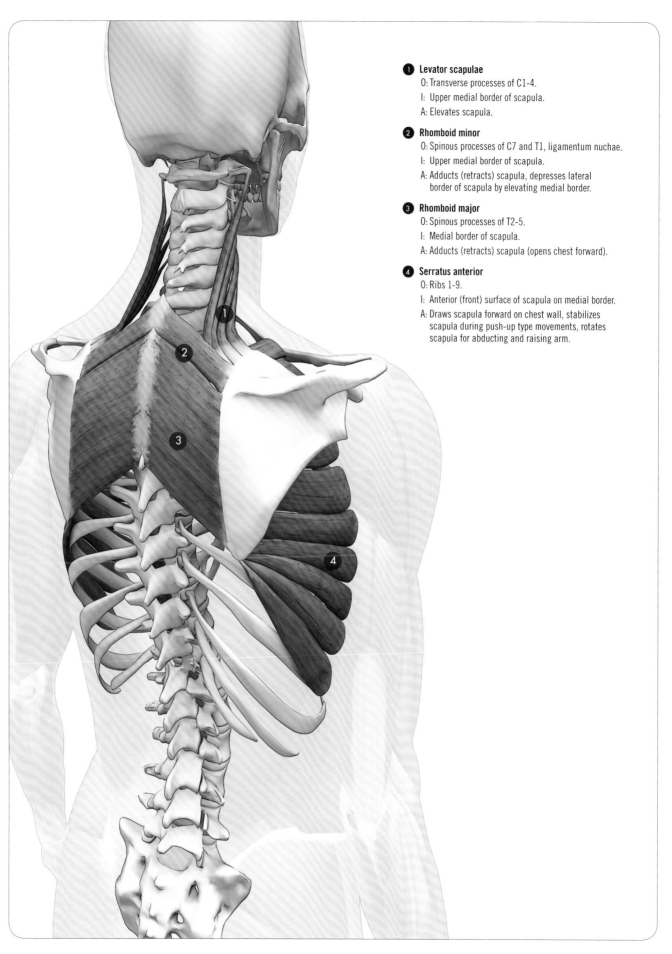

1 **Levator scapulae**
   O: Transverse processes of C1-4.
   I: Upper medial border of scapula.
   A: Elevates scapula.

2 **Rhomboid minor**
   O: Spinous processes of C7 and T1, ligamentum nuchae.
   I: Upper medial border of scapula.
   A: Adducts (retracts) scapula, depresses lateral
       border of scapula by elevating medial border.

3 **Rhomboid major**
   O: Spinous processes of T2-5.
   I: Medial border of scapula.
   A: Adducts (retracts) scapula (opens chest forward).

4 **Serratus anterior**
   O: Ribs 1-9.
   I: Anterior (front) surface of scapula on medial border.
   A: Draws scapula forward on chest wall, stabilizes
       scapula during push-up type movements, rotates
       scapula for abducting and raising arm.

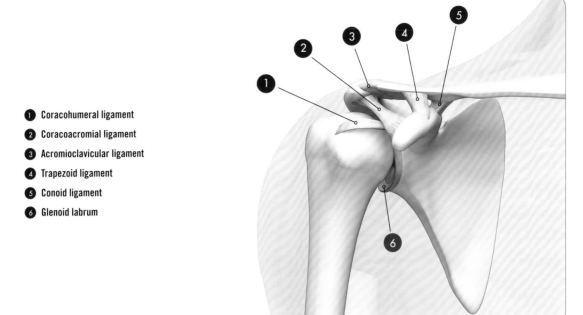

1. Coracohumeral ligament
2. Coracoacromial ligament
3. Acromioclavicular ligament
4. Trapezoid ligament
5. Conoid ligament
6. Glenoid labrum

1. **Supraspinatus**
   O: Supraspinatus fossa of scapula.
   I: Greater tuberosity of humerus.
   A: Initiates abduction of humerus (raising arm to side), stabilizes head of humerus in socket of shoulder joint.

2. **Subscapularis**
   O: Front surface of scapula in subscapular fossa.
   I: Lesser tuberosity of humerus.
   A: Internally rotates humerus, stabilizes head of humerus in socket of shoulder joint.

3. **Teres minor**
   O: Upper part of lateral border of scapula.
   I: Back and lower part of greater tuberosity of humerus.
   A: Externally rotates humerus, stabilizes head of humerus in socket of shoulder joint.

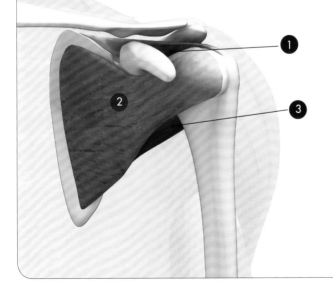

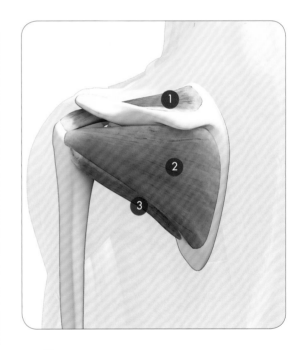

1. **Supraspinatus**
   O: Supraspinatus fossa of scapula.
   I: Greater tuberosity of humerus.
   A: Initiates abduction of humerus (raising arm to side), stabilizes head of humerus in socket of shoulder joint.

2. **Infraspinatus**
   O: Infraspinatus fossa of scapula.
   I: Greater tuberosity of humerus.
   A: Externally rotates shoulder.

3. **Teres minor**
   O: Upper part of lateral border of scapula.
   I: Back and lower part of greater tuberosity of humerus.
   A: Externally rotates humerus, stabilizes head of humerus in socket of shoulder joint.

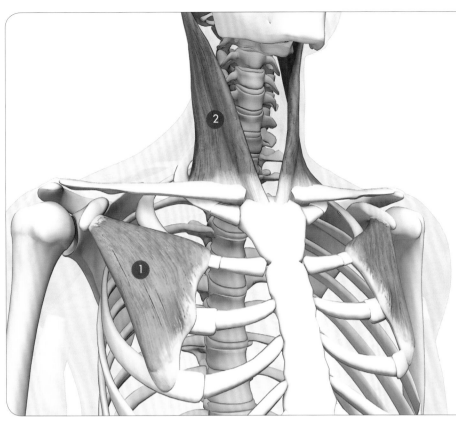

1 Pectoralis minor

O: Front of ribs 3-5.

I: Coracoid process of scapula.

A: Rolls shoulder forward and down (via scapula), lifts ribcage when scapula is stabilized by rhomboids (expands chest) through closed chain contraction.

2 Sternocleidomastoid

O: Sternal head: manubrium of sternum; clavicular head: upper surface of medial third of clavicle.

I: Mastoid process behind and below ear.

A: When both sides contract together flexes neck and tilts head forward; if head is stabilized, lifts upper ribcage during inhalation; contracting one side tilts head to side of muscle, rotates head to face away from muscle.

1 Pectoralis major

O: Sternocostal head: front of manubrium and body of sternum; clavicular head: medial half of clavicle.

I: Outer edge of bicipital groove on upper humerus.

A: Adducts and internally rotates humerus. Sternocostal head draws humerus down and across the body towards opposite hip. Clavicular head forward flexes and internally rotates the humerus, draws humerus across body towards opposite shoulder.

2 Coracobrachialis

O: Coracoid process of scapula.

I: Inner surface of humerus at mid-shaft.

A: Assists pectoralis in adduction of humerus and shoulder.

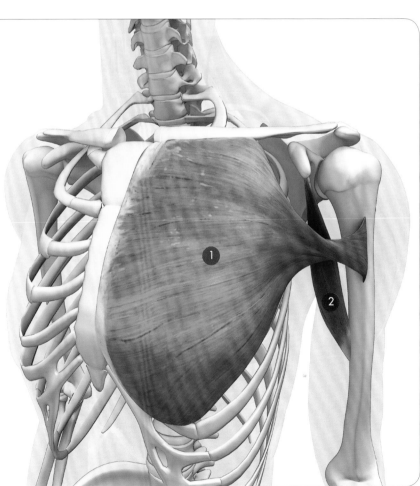

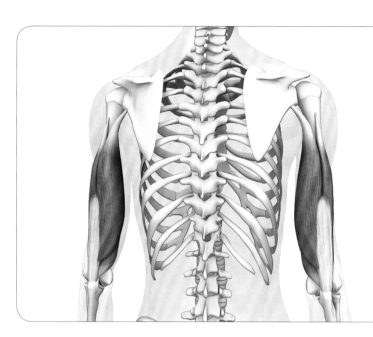

Triceps brachii

O: Long head from infraglenoid tubercle at bottom of shoulder socket; medial and lateral heads from posterior surface of humerus and intermuscular septum.

I: Olecranon process of ulna.

A: Extends elbow, long head moves arm back and adducts it.

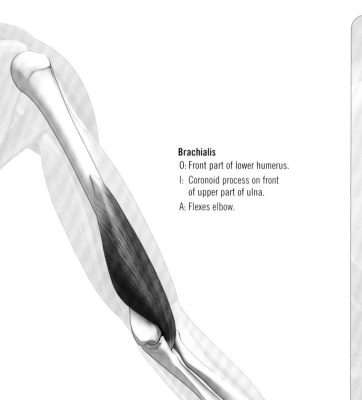

Brachialis

O: Front part of lower humerus.

I: Coronoid process on front of upper part of ulna.

A: Flexes elbow.

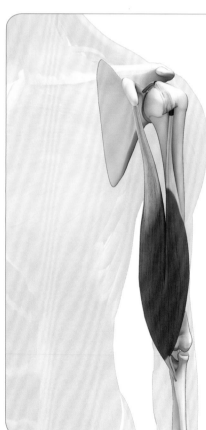

Biceps brachii

O: Long head: upper part of glenoid (socket) of shoulder joint; short head: coracoid process of scapula.

I: Radial tuberosity on upper part of radius.

A: Flexes elbow and supinates forearm.

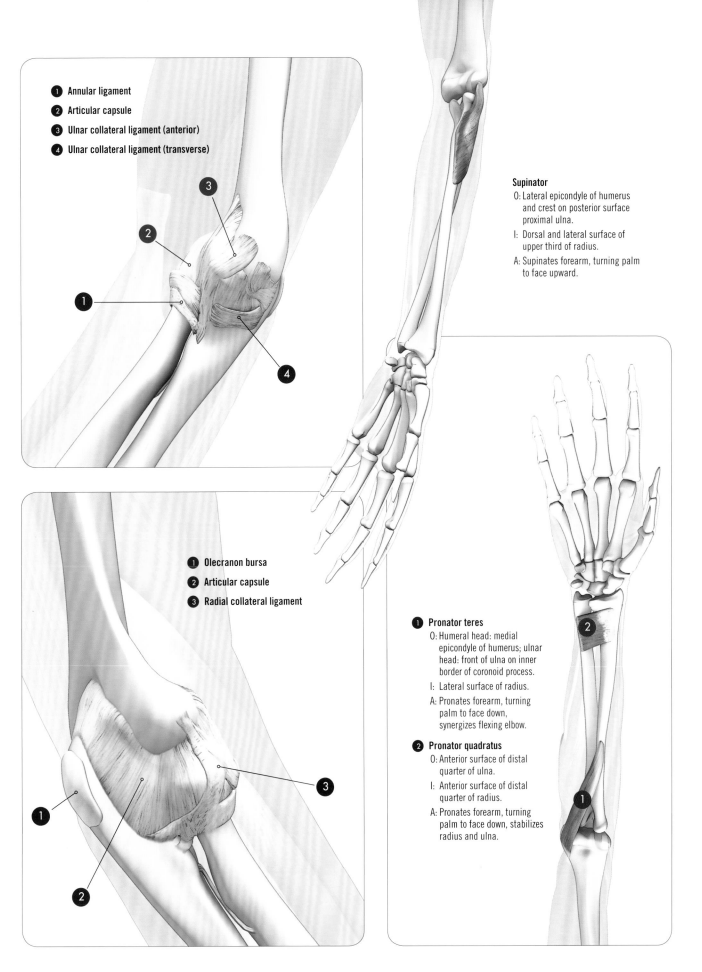

1. Annular ligament
2. Articular capsule
3. Ulnar collateral ligament (anterior)
4. Ulnar collateral ligament (transverse)

Supinator
O: Lateral epicondyle of humerus and crest on posterior surface proximal ulna.
I: Dorsal and lateral surface of upper third of radius.
A: Supinates forearm, turning palm to face upward.

1. Olecranon bursa
2. Articular capsule
3. Radial collateral ligament

1. **Pronator teres**
   O: Humeral head: medial epicondyle of humerus; ulnar head: front of ulna on inner border of coronoid process.
   I: Lateral surface of radius.
   A: Pronates forearm, turning palm to face down, synergizes flexing elbow.

2. **Pronator quadratus**
   O: Anterior surface of distal quarter of ulna.
   I: Anterior surface of distal quarter of radius.
   A: Pronates forearm, turning palm to face down, stabilizes radius and ulna.

1 **Flexor digitorum profundis**

O: Upper two thirds of anterior and medial surface of ulna and interosseous membrane (between radius and ulna).

I: Palmar (anterior) surface of distal phalanges of fingers.

A: Flexes distal phalanges, synergizes flexion of more proximal phalanges and wrist.

2 **Flexor pollicis longus**

O: Anterior surface of mid-shaft of radius, coronoid process of ulna, medial epicondyle.

I: Palmar (anterior) surface of distal phalanx of thumb.

A: Flexes thumb and synergizes flexion of wrist.

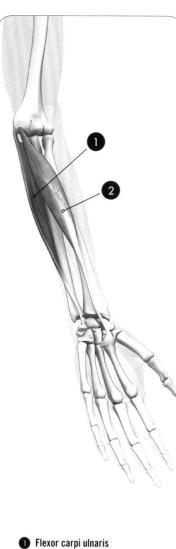

Flexor digitorum superficialis

O: Medial epicondyle, coronoid process of ulna, upper anterior border of radius.

I: Two slips of tendon insert onto either side of middle phalanges of four fingers.

A: Flexes middle phalanges of fingers, synergizes wrist flexion.

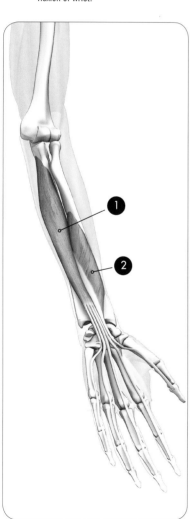

1 **Flexor carpi ulnaris**

O: Medial epicondyle of humerus, medial border and upper two thirds of ulna.

I: Pisiform bone of wrist, base of fifth metacarpal.

A: Flexes and adducts wrist, synergizes elbow flexion.

2 **Flexor carpi radialis**

O: Medial epicondyle of humerus.

I: Base of second metacarpal.

A: Flexes and abducts wrist, synergizes elbow flexion and pronation.

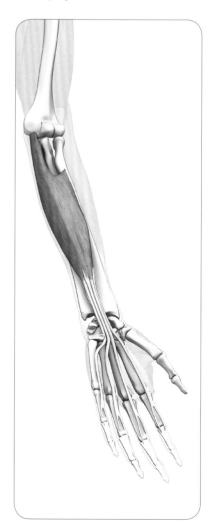

1 **Brachioradialis**

O: Lateral supracondylar ridge of humerus.

I: Lower outside surface of radius, proximal to styloid process.

A: Flexes elbow.

2 **Extensor carpi radialis longus**

O: Lateral supracondylar ridge of humerus.

I: Dorsal surface of base of second metacarpal.

A: Extends and abducts wrist.

3 **Extensor carpi radialis brevis**

O: Lateral epicondyle via common extensor tendon.

I: Dorsal surface of base of third metacarpal.

A: Extends and abducts wrist.

4 **Extensor carpi ulnaris**

O: Lateral epicondyle via common extensor tendon.

I: Base of fifth metacarpal.

A: Extends and adducts wrist.

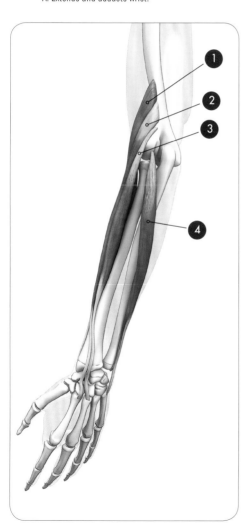

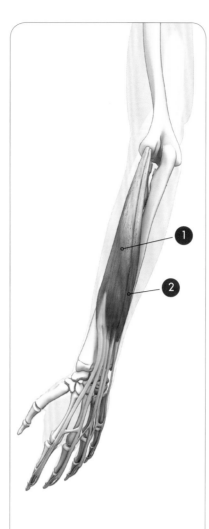

1 **Extensor digitorum**

O: Lateral epicondyle via common extensor tendon.

I: Dorsal surfaces of phalanges of all four fingers.

A: Extends fingers, synergizes finger abduction away from midline.

2 **Extensor digiti minimi**

O: Lateral epicondyle via common extensor tendon.

I: Combines with tendon of extensor digitorum to insert onto dorsum of little finger.

A: Extends little finger.

1 **Abductor pollicis longus**

O: Posterior surface of ulna and radius covering middle third of bones, interosseous membrane.

I: Lateral surface of first metacarpal.

A: Extends and abducts thumb, synergist of forearm supination and wrist flexion.

2 **Extensor pollicis brevis**

O: Posterior surface of distal radius, interosseous membrane.

I: Dorsal surface of base of proximal phalanx of thumb.

A: Extends thumb, synergizes wrist abduction.

3 **Extensor pollicis longus**

O: Posterior surface of middle third of ulna, interosseous membrane.

I: Dorsal surface at base of distal phalanx of thumb.

A: Extends thumb, synergizes wrist extension.

4 **Extensor indicis**

O: Posterior surface of distal ulna, interosseous membrane.

I: Dorsal aponeurosis of index finger, onto proximal phalanx.

A: Extends index finger.

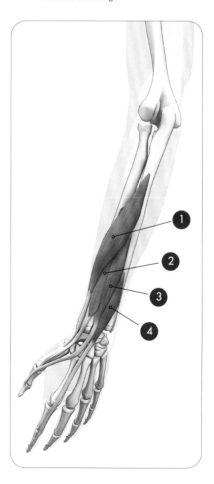

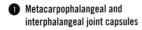

1 Metacarpophalangeal and interphalangeal joint capsules

2 Palmar radiocarpal and intercarpal ligaments

3 Palmar ulnocarpal ligament

1 Transverse metacarpal ligaments

2 Dorsal intercarpal ligaments

3 Dorsal radioulnar ligament

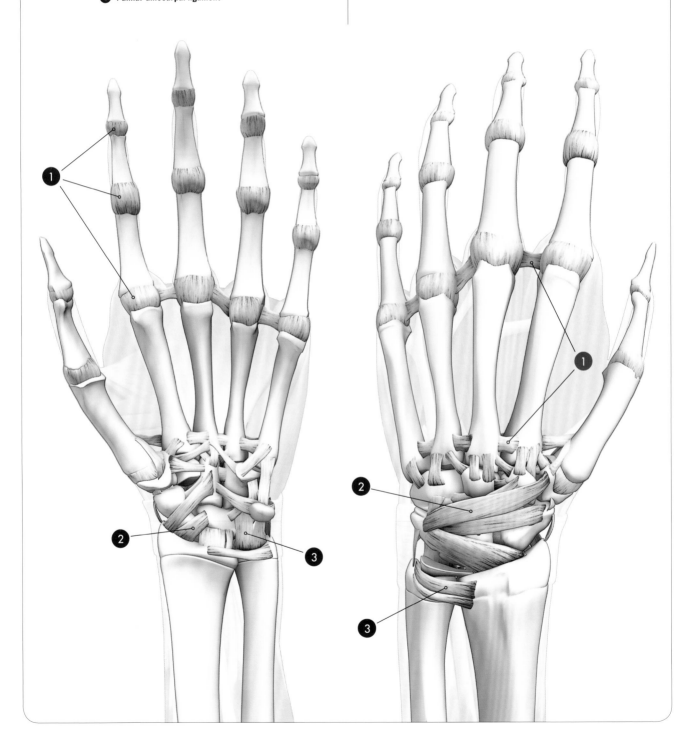

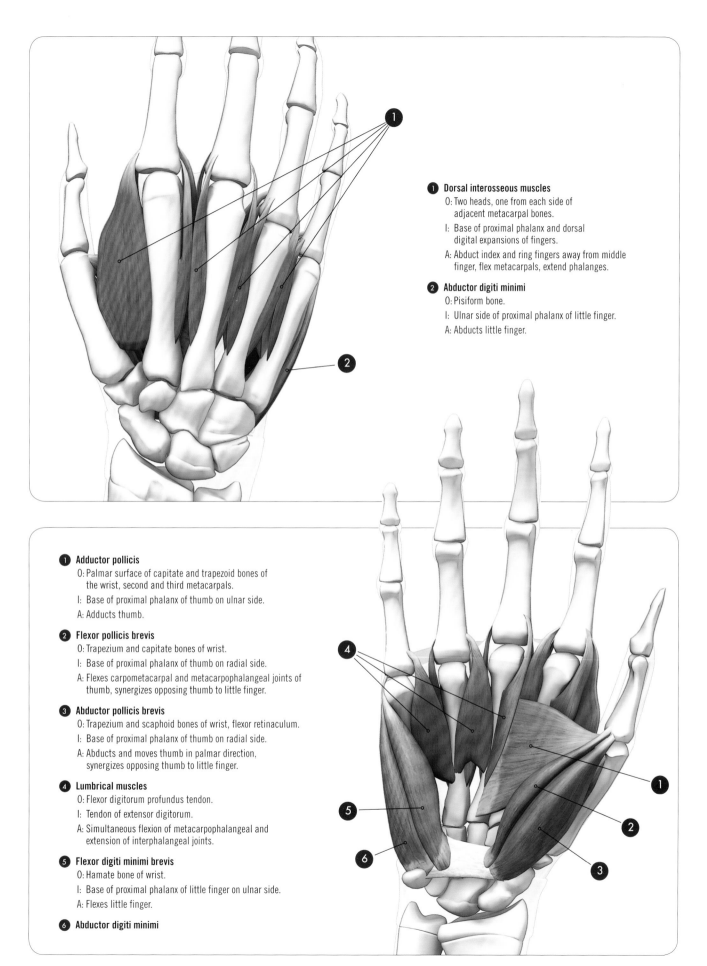

1 **Dorsal interosseous muscles**

O: Two heads, one from each side of adjacent metacarpal bones.

I: Base of proximal phalanx and dorsal digital expansions of fingers.

A: Abduct index and ring fingers away from middle finger, flex metacarpals, extend phalanges.

2 **Abductor digiti minimi**

O: Pisiform bone.

I: Ulnar side of proximal phalanx of little finger.

A: Abducts little finger.

1 **Adductor pollicis**

O: Palmar surface of capitate and trapezoid bones of the wrist, second and third metacarpals.

I: Base of proximal phalanx of thumb on ulnar side.

A: Adducts thumb.

2 **Flexor pollicis brevis**

O: Trapezium and capitate bones of wrist.

I: Base of proximal phalanx of thumb on radial side.

A: Flexes carpometacarpal and metacarpophalangeal joints of thumb, synergizes opposing thumb to little finger.

3 **Abductor pollicis brevis**

O: Trapezium and scaphoid bones of wrist, flexor retinaculum.

I: Base of proximal phalanx of thumb on radial side.

A: Abducts and moves thumb in palmar direction, synergizes opposing thumb to little finger.

4 **Lumbrical muscles**

O: Flexor digitorum profundus tendon.

I: Tendon of extensor digitorum.

A: Simultaneous flexion of metacarpophalangeal and extension of interphalangeal joints.

5 **Flexor digiti minimi brevis**

O: Hamate bone of wrist.

I: Base of proximal phalanx of little finger on ulnar side.

A: Flexes little finger.

6 **Abductor digiti minimi**

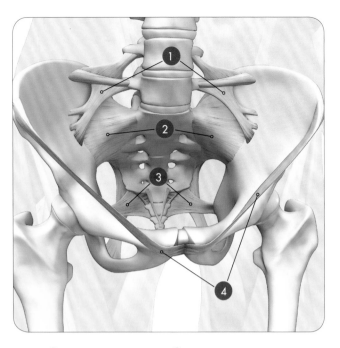

1. Iliolumbar ligament   3. Sacrospinous ligament
2. Sacroiliac ligament   4. Inguinal ligament

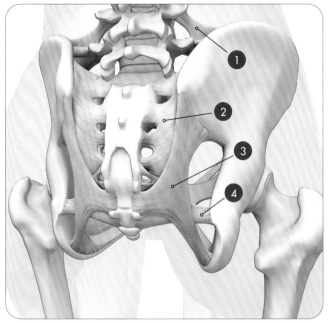

1. Iliolumbar ligament   3. Sacrotuberous ligament
2. Sacroiliac ligament   4. Sacrospinous ligament

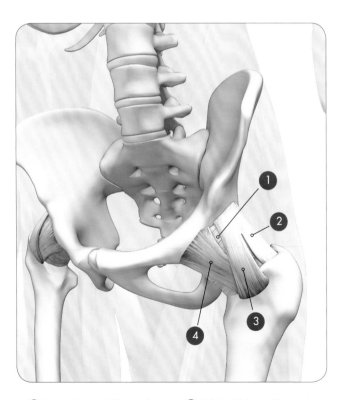

1. Zona orbicularis (hip capsule)   3. Anterior iliofemoral ligament
2. Lateral iliofemoral ligament   4. Pubofemoral ligament

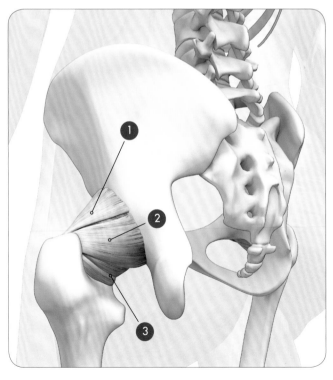

1. Lateral iliofemoral ligament   3. Zona orbicularis (hip capsule)
2. Ischiofemoral ligament

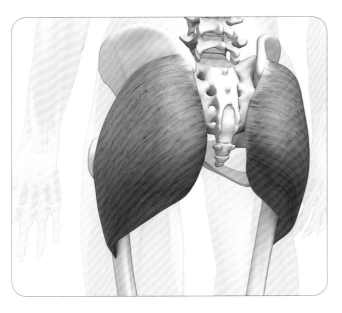

Gluteus maximus

O: Posterolateral surface of ilium and lateral surface of the sacrum.

I: Upper fibers onto iliotibial tract; lower fibers onto gluteal tuberosity.

A: Extends, externally rotates, and stabilizes hip.

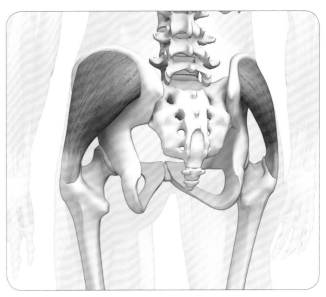

Gluteus medius

O: Outer surface of ilium.

I: Greater trochanter.

A: Abducts hip, anterior fibers internally rotate and flex hip, posterior fibers externally rotate and extend hip.

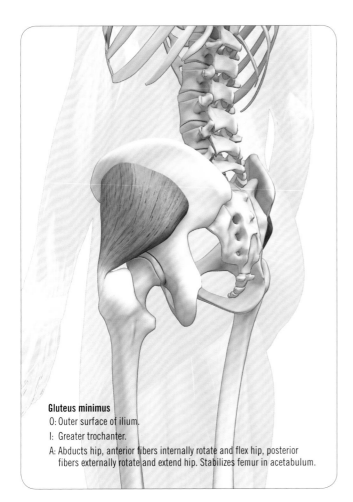

Gluteus minimus

O: Outer surface of ilium.

I: Greater trochanter.

A: Abducts hip, anterior fibers internally rotate and flex hip, posterior fibers externally rotate and extend hip. Stabilizes femur in acetabulum.

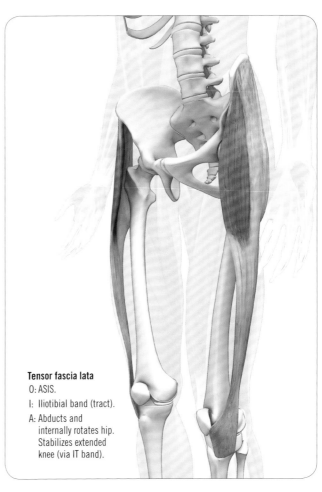

Tensor fascia lata

O: ASIS.

I: Iliotibial band (tract).

A: Abducts and internally rotates hip. Stabilizes extended knee (via IT band).

1 Piriformis

    O: Posterior surface of sacrum.

    I: Greater trochanter.

    A: Externally rotates, abducts, extends, and stabilizes hip.

2 Superior gemellus

    O: Ischial spine.

    I: Greater trochanter.

    A: Externally rotates and adducts hip.

3 Obturator internus

    O: Obturator membrane and ischium.

    I: Greater trochanter.

    A: Externally rotates and adducts hip.

4 Inferior gemellus

    O: Ischial tuberosity.

    I: Greater trochanter.

    A: Externally rotates and adducts hip.

5 Quadratus femoris

    O: Ischial tuberosity.

    I: Intertrochanteric crest.

    A: Externally rotates and adducts hip.

6 Obturator externus

    O: Obturator membrane and ischium.

    I: Greater trochanter.

    A: Externally rotates and adducts hip.

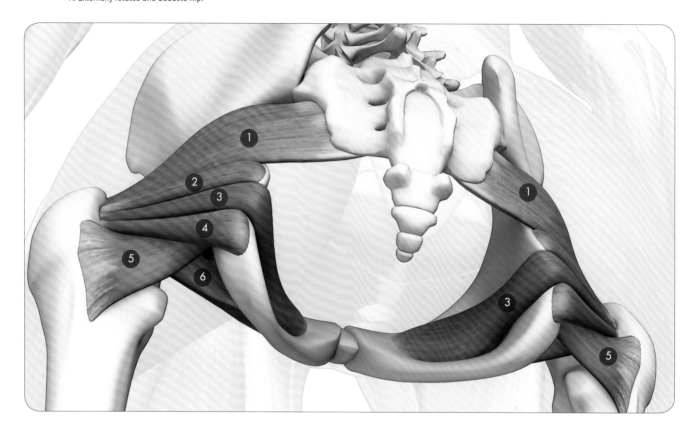

1 Psoas major

    O: T12-L4 vertebral bodies and discs.

    I: Lesser trochanter.

    A: Flexes and externally rotates hip, stabilizes lumbar spine.

2 Iliacus

    O: Inner surface of ilium.

    I: Lesser trochanter.

    A: Flexes and externally rotates hip, with psoas major tilts pelvis forward.

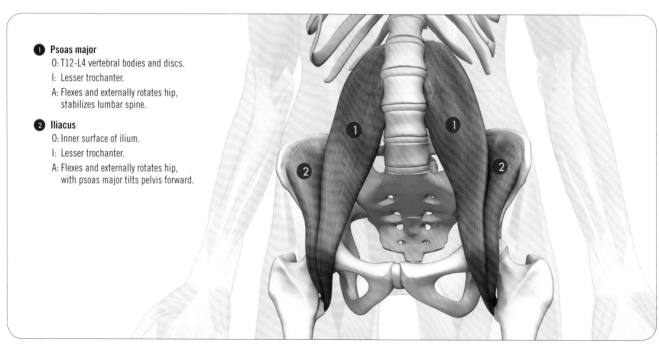

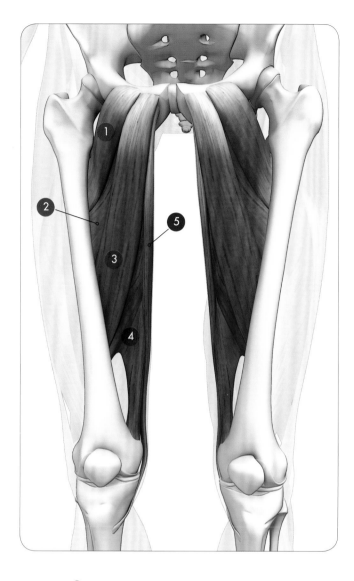

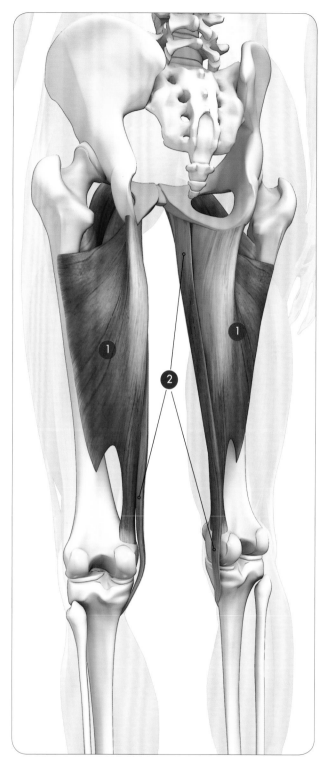

1 Pectineus
O: Pubic bone.
I: Linea aspera of femur.
A: Adducts, externally rotates, and synergizes femur flexion.

2 Adductor brevis
O: Pubic bone.
I: Linea aspera of femur.
A: Adducts and flexes femur, stabilizes pelvis.

3 Adductor longus
O: Pubic bone.
I: Linea aspera of femur.
A: Adducts and flexes femur, stabilizes pelvis.

4 Adductor magnus
O: Pubic bone and ischial tuberosity.
I: Linea aspera and medial epicondyle of femur.
A: Adducts, externally rotates, and extends femur.

5 Gracilis
O: Pubic bone.
I: Medial tibia.
A: Adducts and flexes hip, flexes and internally rotates knee.

1 Adductor magnus

2 Gracilis

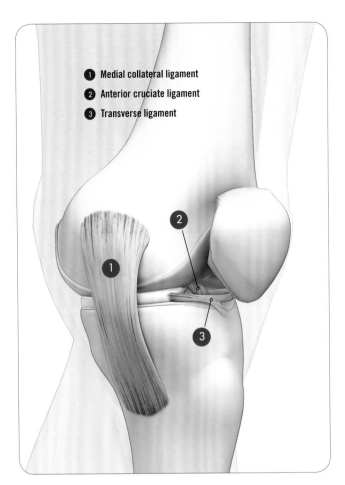

1 Medial collateral ligament
2 Anterior cruciate ligament
3 Transverse ligament

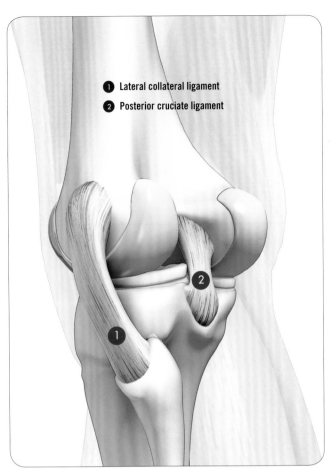

1 Lateral collateral ligament
2 Posterior cruciate ligament

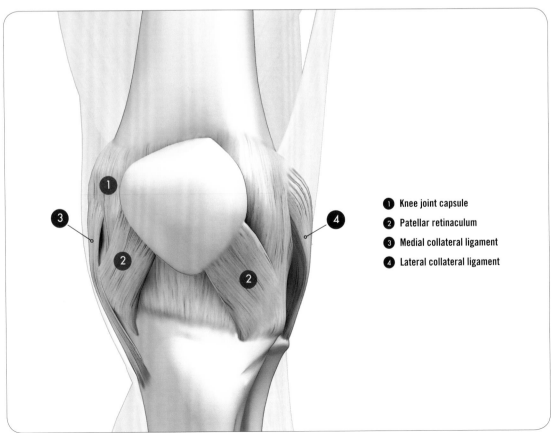

1 Knee joint capsule
2 Patellar retinaculum
3 Medial collateral ligament
4 Lateral collateral ligament

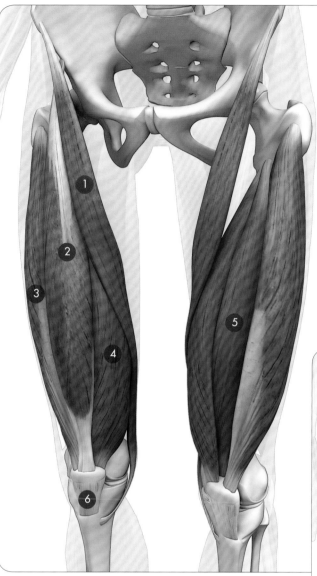

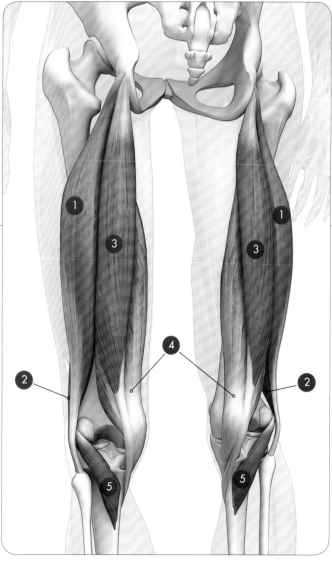

① **Sartorius**
   O: ASIS.
   I: Pes anserinus of medial tibia.
   A: Flexes, abducts, and externally rotates hip; flexes and internally rotates knee.

② **Rectus femoris**
   O: ASIS.
   I: Anterior tibia via patellar tendon.
   A: Flexes hip, tilts pelvis forward, extends knee.

③ **Vastus lateralis**
   O: Lateral femur.
   I: Anterior tibia via patellar tendon.
   A: Extends knee.

④ **Vastus medialis**
   O: Medial femur.
   I: Anterior tibia via patellar tendon.
   A: Extends knee.

⑤ **Vastus intermedius**
   O: Anterior femur.
   I: Anterior tibia via patellar tendon.
   A: Extends knee.

⑥ **Patellar tendon**

① **Biceps femoris long head**
   O: Ischial tuberosity.
   I: Fibular head.
   A: Extends hip, flexes and externally rotates knee.

② **Biceps femoris short head**
   O: Posterior surface of femur.
   I: Fibular head.
   A: Extends hip, flexes and externally rotates knee.

③ **Semitendinosus**
   O: Ischial tuberosity.
   I: Pes anserinus of medial tibia.
   A: Extends hip, flexes and internally rotates knee.

④ **Semimembranosus**
   O: Ischial tuberosity.
   I: Back of medial tibial condyle.
   A: Extends hip, flexes and internally rotates knee.

⑤ **Popliteus**
   O: Lateral femoral condyle.
   I: Posterior surface of tibia, below knee joint.
   A: Flexes and internally rotates knee.

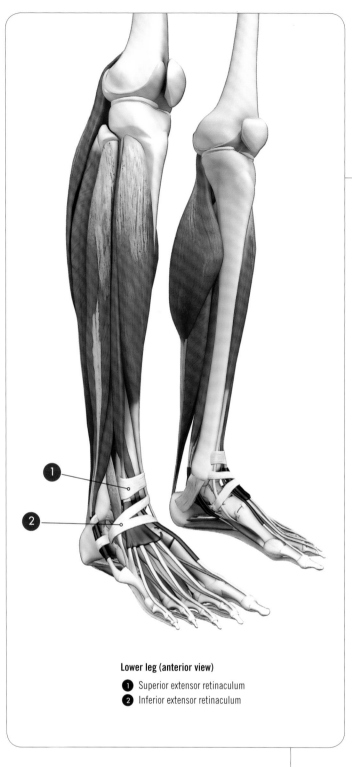

Lower leg (anterior view)

1 Superior extensor retinaculum
2 Inferior extensor retinaculum

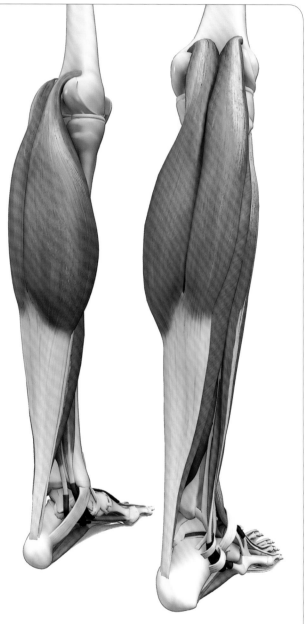

Lower leg (posterior view)

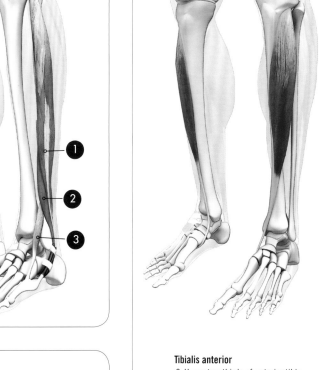

1 **Peroneus longus**

O: Head and proximal two thirds of lateral fibula.

I: Base of first metacarpal and medial cuneiform.

A: Plantar flexes ankle and everts subtalar joint, supports transverse arch of foot.

2 **Peroneus brevis**

O: Distal half of lateral surface of fibula, intermuscular membrane.

I: Base of fifth metatarsal.

A: Plantar flexes ankle and everts subtalar joint.

3 **Peroneus tertius**

O: Front of distal fibula.

I: Base of fifth metatarsal.

A: Dorsiflexes ankle and everts subtalar joint.

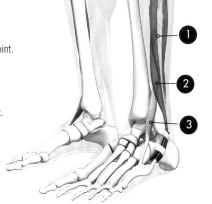

Tibialis anterior

O: Upper two thirds of anterior tibia and interosseous membrane.

I: Medial cuneiform, base of first metatarsal.

A: Dorsiflexes ankle, inverts subtalar joint.

1 **Gastrocnemius**

O: Medial head from medial epicondyle of femur; lateral head from lateral epicondyle.

I: Calcaneous via Achilles tendon.

A: Plantar flexes and inverts ankle, flexes knee.

2 **Soleus**

O: Posterior surface of head and neck of fibula.

I: Calcaneous via Achilles tendon.

A: Plantar flexes ankle, inverts subtalar joint.

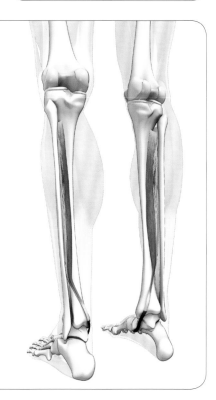

Tibialis posterior

O: Interosseous membrane between tibia and fibula.

I: Navicular, cuneiform bones, and second through fourth metatarsals.

A: Plantar flexes ankle, inverts subtalar joint, and supports longitudinal and transverse foot arches.

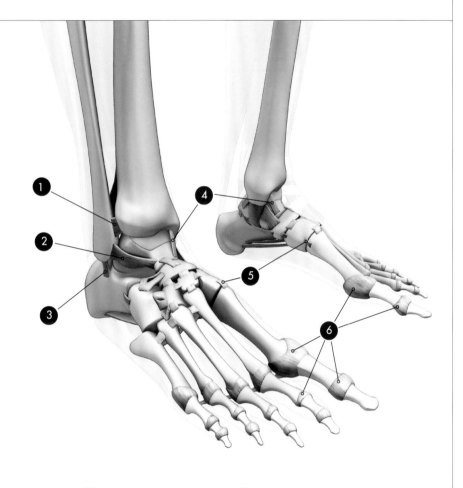

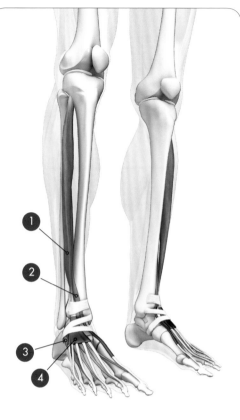

1 Extensor digitorum longus

   O: Lateral tibial condyle, fibular head, interosseous membrane.

   I: Dorsal aponeurosis and bases of the distal phalanges of second through fifth toes.

   A: Dorsiflexes ankle, everts subtalar joint, and extends metatarsophalangeal and interphalangeal joints of toes.

2 Extensor hallucis longus

   O: Medial surface of fibula, interosseous membrane.

   I: Dorsal aponeurosis and base of distal phalanx of big toe.

   A: Dorsiflexes ankle, everts subtalar joint, and extends big toe.

3 Extensor digitorum brevis

   O: Dorsal surface of calcaneous.

   I: Dorsal aponeurosis and bases of middle phalanges of second through fourth toes.

   A: Extends metatarsophalangeal and proximal interphalangeal joints of second through fourth toes.

4 Extensor tendons sheath

1 Anterior tibiofibular ligament   **4** Anterior tibiotalar ligament

2 Anterior talofibular ligament   **5** Dorsal metatarsal ligaments

3 Calcaneofibular ligament   **6** Interphalangeal joint capsules

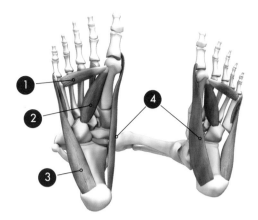

1 **Adductor hallucis (transverse head)**

O: Metatarsophalangeal joints of third through fifth toes.

I: Base of proximal phalanx of big toe via sesamoid.

A: Adducts and flexes big toe, supports transverse foot arch.

2 **Adductor hallucis (oblique head)**

O: Bases of second through fourth metatarsals, lateral cuneiform, and cuboid.

I: Base of proximal phalanx of big toe via sesamoid.

A: Adducts and flexes big toe, supports longitudinal foot arch.

3 **Abductor digiti minimi**

O: Calcaneous, plantar aponeurosis.

I: Base of proximal phalanx of little toe.

A: Flexes metatarsophalangeal joint and abducts little toe, supports longitudinal foot arch.

4 **Abductor hallucis**

O: Calcaneous, plantar aponeurosis.

I: Base of proximal phalanx of big toe.

A: Flexes and abducts big toe, supports longitudinal foot arch.

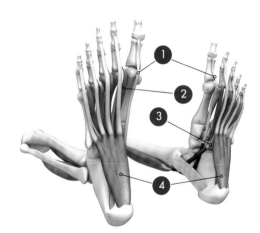

1 **Flexor hallucis longus**

O: Posterior surface of fibula, interosseous membrane.

I: Base of distal phalanx of big toe.

A: Plantar flexes ankle, inverts subtalar joint, flexes big toe, supports longitudinal foot arch.

2 **Lumbrical muscles**

O: Medial borders of flexor digitorum longus tendons.

I: Dorsal aponeurosis of second through fifth toes.

A: Flexes metatarsophalangeal and extends interphalangeal joints of second through fifth toes, adducts toe.

3 **Flexor digitorum longus**

O: Posterior surface of tibia.

I: Bases of distal phalanges of second through fifth toes.

A: Plantar flexes ankle, inverts subtalar joint, plantar flexes toes.

4 **Flexor digitorum brevis**

O: Calcaneous, plantar aponeurosis.

I: Middle phalanges of second through fifth toes.

A: Flexes toes, supports longitudinal foot arch.

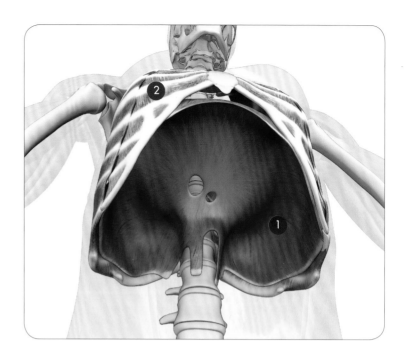

1 Diaphragm

O: Lower margin of costal arch, posterior surface of xiphoid process of sternum, arcuate ligament of aorta, L1-3 vertebral bodies.

I: Central tendon.

A: Primary muscle of respiration, aids in compressing abdomen.

2 Intercostals

O: Internal intercostals from surface of upper margin of rib; external intercostals from lower margin of rib.

I: Internals insert on lower margin of next higher rib; externals insert on upper margin of next lower rib.

A: Internal intercostals lower ribs during exhalation; externals raise ribs during inhalation.

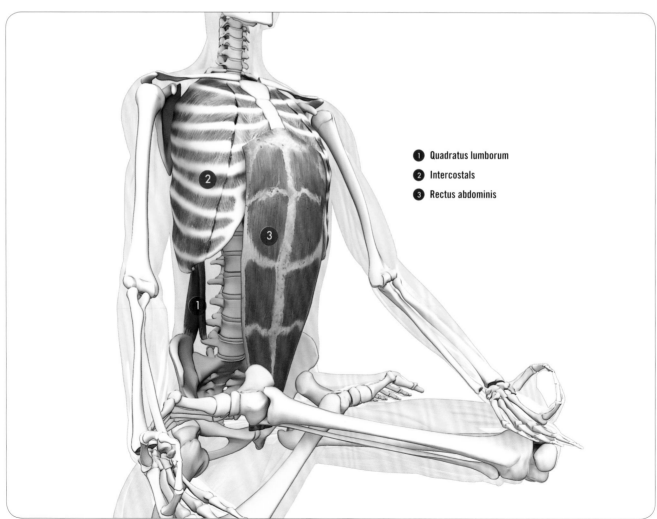

1 Quadratus lumborum

2 Intercostals

3 Rectus abdominis

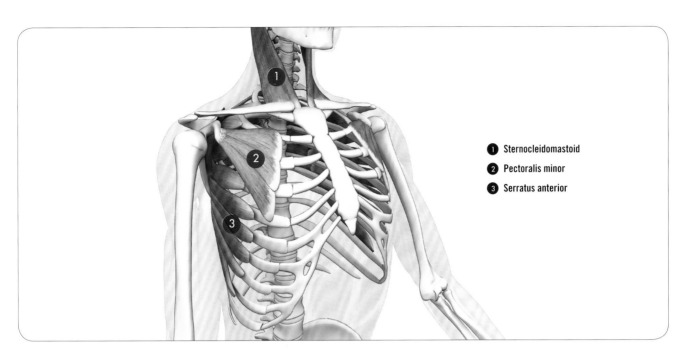

1 Sternocleidomastoid
2 Pectoralis minor
3 Serratus anterior

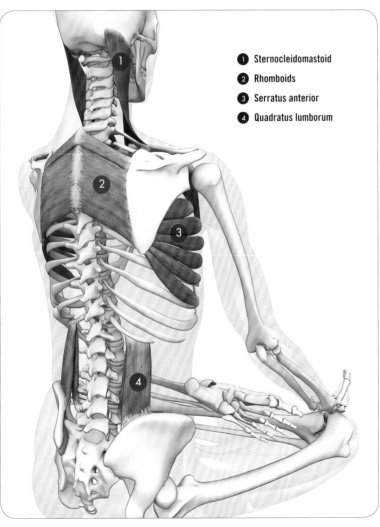

1 Sternocleidomastoid
2 Rhomboids
3 Serratus anterior
4 Quadratus lumborum

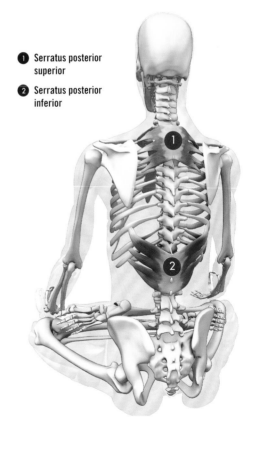

1 Serratus posterior superior
2 Serratus posterior inferior

INDEX OF MUSCLES
AND LIGAMENTS

GLOSSARY OF TERMS

Abduction Moving away from the midline.

Accessory muscles of breathing Muscles that attach to the ribcage and thorax that can be used to augment the action of the diaphragm for inhalation and exhalation. These include the rhomboids, pectorals, quadratus lumborum, sternocleidomastoid, and intercostals (among others).

Active insufficiency A condition in which a muscle is shortened or lengthened to a point where it can no longer effectively move a joint. For example, in Kurmasana the hips are fully flexed and so the psoas muscle is shortened to a point where it cannot effectively flex the hips further. At such times, other parts of the body must be used for leverage, such as the arms under the knees.

Adduction Moving toward the midline.

Agonist The muscle that contracts to produce a certain action about a joint (sometimes referred to as the prime mover). For example, the brachialis contracts to flex the elbow joint.

Alveoli Sac-like spherical structures with thin membrane-like walls through which gas exchange occurs in the lungs.

Anatomy The study of the structure of living things. Musculoskeletal anatomy studies the bones, ligaments, muscles, and tendons.

Antagonist The muscle that opposes the action of the agonist muscle and produces the opposite action about a joint. For example, the hamstrings are the antagonists to the quadriceps for extending the knee.

Anteversion Tilting forward.

Aponeurosis A fibrous thickening of fascia that forms the attachment for muscles. For example, the abdominal muscles attach to the linea alba, an aponeurotic thickening at the front of the abdomen.

Appendicular skeleton Composed of the shoulder (pectoral girdle) and upper extremities and pelvis and lower extremities.

Asana Sanskrit term for body position in yoga (yogasana).

Autonomic nervous system Part of the nervous system that functions largely unconsciously to control breathing, heart rate, blood pressure, digestion, perspiration, and other functions. It is divided into the sympathetic (fight or flight) and parasympathetic (rest and digest) nervous systems.

Axial skeleton Composed of the skull, spine, and ribcage.

Bandha Sanskrit term referring to binding, locking, or stabilizing. Co-activating muscle groups can be used to form bandhas in yoga postures.

Biomechanics The application of mechanical physics to the body. For example, contracting the biceps flexes the elbow joint.

Carpals The bones of the wrist, including the scaphoid, lunate, triquetrum, hamate, capitate, trapezoid, and trapezium.

Center of gravity The center of an object's weight distribution and at which point an object is in balance.

Center of gravity projection An extension of the force of gravity downward and away from the body. For example, in Warrior III the center of gravity is projected out through the arms and the back leg, balancing the pose.

Chakra Wheel-like centers or concentrations of energy within the subtle body. They may correspond to collections of nerves such as the lumbosacral plexus (for the first and second chakras).

Closed chain contraction/movement The origin of the muscle moves and the insertion remains stationary. For example, the psoas contracts to flex the trunk in Trikonasana.

Co-contraction/co-activation Simultaneously contracting agonist and antagonist muscles to stabilize a joint. For example, co-activating the peroneus longus and brevis and the tibialis posterior muscles stabilizes the ankle joint.

Core muscles Composed of the transversus abdominis, internal and external obliques, rectus abdominis, erector spinae, psoas, gluteus maximus, and pelvic diaphragm.

Drishti Sanskrit term for focus of vision or gaze.

Eccentric contraction The muscle generates tension (contracts) while lengthening.

Erector spinae The group of three deep back muscles that run parallel to the spinal column, including the spinalis, longissimus, and iliocostalis muscles.

Eversion Rotating the sole of the foot (via the ankle) away from the midline of the body. This is associated with pronation (internal rotation) of the forefoot.

Extension Joint movement that increases space and distance between skeletal segments, bringing them farther apart.

Facilitated stretching A powerful method of stretching in which the muscle is first taken out to its full length and then contracted for several moments. This stimulates the Golgi tendon organ and produces the "relaxation response," causing the muscle to relax and lengthen. It is also known as PNF.

Fascia Connective tissue that surrounds, separates, and binds muscles to each other. This can also form an aponeurosis for muscle attachment.

Flexion Joint movement that decreases space between skeletal segments and draws them closer together.

Floating ribs Five pairs of ribs that articulate posteriorly with the vertebrae and attach to the costal cartilage anteriorly.

Forefoot The region of the foot distal to the midfoot. It is composed of the metatarsal and phalangeal bones (and their corresponding joints). Motion includes toe flexion and extension and deepening of the foot arches.

Glenohumeral joint Ball and socket synovial joint where the head (ball) of the humerus articulates with the glenoid fossa (socket) of the scapula.

Golgi tendon organ A sensory receptor located at the muscle-tendon junction that detects changes in tension. This information is conveyed to the central nervous system, which then signals the muscle to relax, providing "slack" in the muscle. This protects against the tendon being torn from the bone. The Golgi tendon organ is central to PNF or facilitated stretching.

Hindfoot Typically refers to the calcaneous and talus bones. The joint for the hindfoot is the subtalar joint, which is responsible for everting and inverting the foot. For example, the hindfoot is inverted in the back leg in Warrior I.

Iliotibial tract Fibrous fascial structure that runs on the outside of the thigh and blends into the lateral portion of the knee capsule. This forms the attachment for the tensor fascia lata and part of the gluteus maximus muscles.

Impingement Narrowing or encroachment of the space between two bones. It can cause inflammation and pain. For example, a nerve root can become impinged by a herniated intervertebral disc. You can also have impingement between the humeral head and the acromion, causing pain in the shoulder.

Insertion The distal site where a muscle attaches to a bone (via a tendon), usually farther from the midline of the body and more mobile than the muscle origin at its opposite end.

Inversion Rotating the sole of the foot towards the midline of the body (turning it inward). This is associated with supination (external rotation) of the forefoot.

Isometric contraction The muscle generates tension but does not shorten, and the bones do not move.

Isotonic contraction The muscle shortens while maintaining constant tension through a range of motion.

Kriya Sanskrit term for action or activity.

Leverage Creating a mechanical advantage based on the length of the lever. For example, placing the hand on the outside of the foot in Parivrtta Trikonasana uses the length of the arm for leverage to turn the body.

Line of action A line through which forces act or are directed within the body. For example, there is a line of action extending from the tips of the fingers to the heel in Utthita Parsvakonasana.

Metacarpals The intermediate region of the hand between the carpus (wrist) and the fingers, i.e., the five bones of the palms of the hands.

Midfoot The intermediate region of the foot between the hindfoot and forefoot. It is composed of the navicular, the cuboid, and three cuneiform bones. Motion includes contribution to supination and pronation of the forefoot.

Mudra Sanskrit term for seal; similar to a bandha. It is often performed with the hands by bringing the fingertips together in a specific way. Other mudras are created by combining bandhas throughout the body.

Muscle spindle A sensory receptor within the muscle belly that detects changes in length and tension in the muscle. This information is conveyed to the central nervous system which can then signal the muscle to contract to resist stretching. This reflex protects against tearing the muscle.

Open chain contraction/movement The insertion of the muscle moves and the origin remains stationary. For example, the deltoids contract to lift the arms in Warrior II.

Origin The proximal site where a muscle attaches to a bone (via a tendon), usually closer to the midline of the body and less mobile than the muscle insertion on the bone at its opposite end.

Parivrtta Revolving, twisted, or turning version of a pose. For example, Parivrtta Trikonasana is the revolving version of Trikonasana (Triangle Pose).

Pelvic girdle The ilium, ischium, pubic bones, and pubic symphysis.

Physiology The study of the functional processes of living things. Most physiological processes take place unconsciously but can be influenced by the conscious mind. Examples include breathing and facilitated stretching.

PNF Proprioceptive neuromuscular facilitation. Also known as *facilitated stretching*. (See facilitated stretching.)

Posterior kinetic chain Composed of a group of interconnecting ligaments, tendons, and muscles on the back of the body. Includes the hamstrings, gluteus maximus, erector spinae, trapezius, latissimus, and posterior deltoids.

Pranayama Yogic art of controlling the breath.

Prime mover The muscle that contracts to directly produce a desired movement. For example, the quadriceps contracts to extend the knee joint. The term is sometimes used interchangeably with 'agonist muscle.'

Radial deviation Tilting the hand toward the index-finger side or away from the midline of the body.

Reciprocal inhibition A phenomenon whereby the brain signals an agonist muscle to contract, and a simultaneous inhibitory signal is sent to the antagonist muscle, causing it to relax. This physiological process takes place unconsciously.

Retroversion Tilting backward.

Rotation Joint movement around a longitudinal axis. For example, we externally rotate the humerus bones (longitudinal axis) to turn the palms to face up in Savasana.

Scapulohumeral rhythm Simultaneous movements at the glenohumeral and scapulothoracic joints that function together to abduct and flex the shoulders. For example, scapulohumeral rhythm takes place when we raise the arms overhead in Urdhva Hastasana.

Shoulder girdle The clavicles and scapulae.

Synergist A muscle that assists and fine-tunes the action of the agonist or prime mover. It can be used to produce the same action, although generally not as efficiently. For example, the pectineus muscle synergizes the psoas in flexing the hip joint.

True ribs Seven pairs of ribs that articulate posteriorly with the vertebrae and anteriorly with the sternum.

Ulnar deviation Tilting the hand toward the little-finger side or midline of the body.

SANSKRIT PRONUNCIATION AND POSE INDEX

Sanskrit	Pronunciation	Pages
Adho Mukha Svanasana	[AH-doh MOO-kah shvah-NAHS-anna]	**27**
Adho Mukha Vrksasana	[ah-doh moo-kah vriks-SHAHS-anna]	**100**
Astavakrasana	[ahsh-tah-vah-krahs-anna]	**75**
Bakasana	[bahk-AHS-anna]	7, 17, **47**, 84, 90
Balasana	[bahl-AHS-anna]	168
Bhujapidasana	[boo-jah-pee-DAHS-anna]	8, **68**, 75
Chaturanga Dandasana	[chaht-tour-ANG-ah don-DAHS-anna]	**34**, 62, 70, 76, 80, 102, 110
Eka Pada Bakasana I	[A-kah pah-dah bahk-AHS-anna]	**82**
Eka Pada Bakasana II	[A-kah pah-dah bahk-AHS-anna]	7, **54**
Eka Pada Sarvangasana	[A-kah pah-dah sar-van-GAHS-anna]	16, 19, **148**, 156
Eka Pada Sirsasana	[A-kah pah-dah shear-SHAHS-anna]	13, **133**
Garudasana	[gah-roo-dahs-anna]	109, 110
Gomukhasana	[go-moo-KAHS-anna]	109
Halasana	[hah-LAHS-anna]	6, 7, 142, 150, **156**, 164
Hanumanasana	[hah-new-mahn-AHS-anna]	84, 102, 134, 150
Kurmasana	[koohr-MAH-sah-nah]	15, 54, 56, 62, 64, 68, 70, 76, 158, 164, 15
Marichyasana III	[mar-ee-chee-AHS-anna]	76, 164
Paschimottanasana	[POSH-ee-moh-tan-AHS-anna]	54, 158
Parsva Bakasana	[PARSH-vah bahk-AHS-anna]	**90**, 17
Parsva Halasana	[PARSH-vah hah-LAHS-anna]	**162**
Parsva Sirsasana	[PARSH-vah shear-SHAHS-anna]	**125**
Parsvottanasana	[pars-VOH-tahn-AHS-ahna]	134, 150
Pincha Mayurasana	[pin-cha my-your-AHS-anna]	**109**
Prasarita Padottanasana	[pra-sa-REE-tah pah-doh-tahn-AHS-anna]	70
Purvottanasana	[purvo-tan AHS-ahna]	142
Savasana	[shah-VAHS-anna]	169
Salamba Sarvangasana	[sar-van-GAHS-anna]	8, 9, **140**, 148, 150
Setu Bandha Sarvangasana	[SET-too BAHN-dah sar-van-GAHS-anna]	142
Sirsasana	[shear-SHAHS-anna]	11, **116**, 126, 134, 139
Supta Padangusthasana, Bent-Knee Version	[soup-TAH pod-ang-goosh-TAHS-anna]	76

SANSKRIT PRONUNCIATION AND POSE INDEX CONTINUED

Sanskrit	Pronunciation	Pages
Tadasana	[tah-DAS-anna}	70
Tittibhasana	[ti-tee-BAHS-anna]	15, **62**, 68
Triang Mukhaikapada Paschimottanasana	[tree-AWN-guh moo-KA-eh-ka-paw-duh POSH-ee-moh-tun-AWS-anna]	54, 56
Upavistha Konasana	[oo-pah-VEESH-tah cone-AHS-anna]	164
Uttanasana	[OOT-tan-AHS-anna]	34, 48, 56, 70, 84, 118
Vasisthasana	[vah-sish-TAHS-ahna]	**41**
Viparita Karani	[vip-par-ee-tah car-AHN-ee]	169

Other Sanskrit Terms	Pronunciation	Pages
Asana	[AHS-anna]	——
Ashtanga	[UHSSH-TAWN-gah]	——
Bandha	[bahn-dah]	16, 19
Chakra	[CHUHK-ruh]	106, 123, 161, 167
Drishti	[dr-ISH-tee]	——
Hatha	[huh-tuh]	——
Jalandhara Bandha	[jah-lahn-DHA-rah bahn-dah]	——
Kriya	[kr-EE-yah]	125, 162
Mudra	[MOO-drah]	——
Mula Bandha	[moo-lah bahn-dah]	34, 54, 92
Namasté	[nah-moss-te (*te* rhymes with *day*)]	——
Pranayama	[PRAH-nah-yama]	——
Udyana Bandha	[oo-dee-YAH-nah BAHN-dah]	——
Ujjayi	[oo-jy (*jy* rhymes with *pie*)-ee]	——
Vinyasa	[vin-YAH-sah]	27, 28, 34
Yoga	[YO-gah]	——

ENGLISH POSE INDEX

CONTRIBUTORS

CHRIS MACIVOR—a self-taught computer expert and digital artist—is the Technical Director for Bandha Yoga and Illustrator of the bestselling series, *The Key Muscles of Yoga* and *The Key Poses of Yoga*. He is a graduate of Etobicoke School of the Arts, Sheridan College, and Seneca College. With a background in dance and traditional art, as well as computer graphics and animation, Chris considers himself to be equally artistic and technical in nature. Working with Dr. Long on the Scientific Keys book series, he has digitally reproduced the biomechanical perfection of the human body. With a keen eye for subtle lighting and a passion for excellence in his art, Chris successfully brings his imagery to life.

KURT LONG, BFA, is an award-winning fine artist and anatomical illustrator who contributed the front and back cover illustrations. He is a graduate of the University of Pennsylvania and has studied at the Pennsylvania Academy of Fine Arts and the Art Students League of New York. Kurt resides in Philadelphia with his wife and two sons. For information on commissions and to see more of his work, go to www.KurtLong.net.

STEWART THOMAS contributed the Sanskrit calligraphy and the special hand-painted border for the Bandha Yoga Codex. He is an award-winning artist, calligrapher, printmaker and designer. A graduate of Haverford College and the University of the Arts in Philadelphia, he serves as Creative Director of Florida's Eden, a regional alliance working for a sustainable future for North Florida, and produces art at his own Palmstone Studio (www.palmstone.com).

ERYN KIRKWOOD, MA, RYT 200, graduated from Carleton University with a Master's Degree in English Literature. She left a corporate career as Managing Editor at the Canadian Medical Association to dedicate her life to the study, practice, and teaching of yoga. Eryn is the Chief Editor at Bandha Yoga and maintains an award-winning Blog. She offers alignment-focused yoga classes in Ottawa, Canada, and can be reached at www.BarrhavenYoga.com.

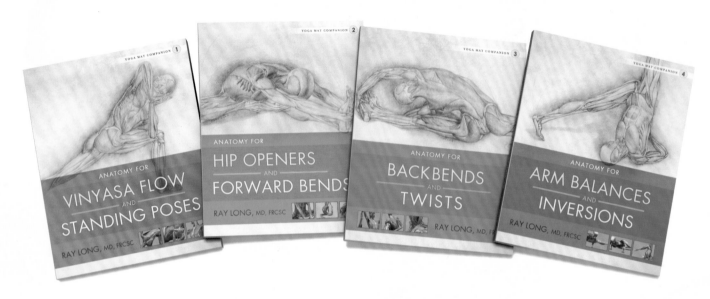

ALSO FROM BANDHA YOGA

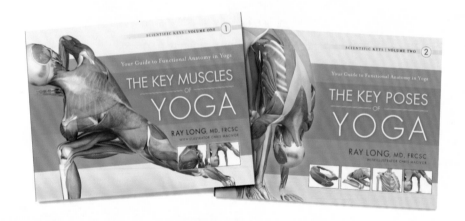

www.BandhaYoga.com